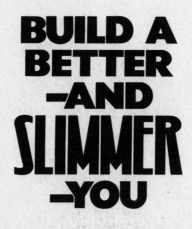

BUILD A BETTER BETTER —AND SLIMMER —YOU

BUILD A BETTER —AND SLIMMER —YOU

JEAN ALLEN & EMILY S. MIX

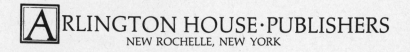

ARLINGTON HOUSE·PUBLISHERS
NEW ROCHELLE, NEW YORK

Manufactured in the United States of America

Library of Congress Cataloging in Publication Data

Allen, Jean, 1932-

   Build a better—and slimmer—you.

   1. Obesity—Psychological aspects. 2. Reducing
diets—Recipes. 3. Reducing exercises. I. Mix,
Emily S., joint author. II. Title.
RC628.A44   613.2′5   76-58039
ISBN 0-87000-369-0

Where most of us end up, there
is no knowing; but the hellbent
get where they are going.
JAMES THURBER

To
O. F.

ACKNOWLEDGMENTS

We wish to thank Ray and Gini who helped us want to rebuild ourselves; Drs. Stuelke, Nelius, and Musante, and all fellow dieters who gave us the bricks with which to build; Norma, Annie, Pitts, and the others for their insight and encouragement to share our building experience.

Our appreciation also to our families and friends, with special thanks to Ed, Mit, Alice, and Ted, who helped us persevere throughout our building, for their faith, trust, love, and unending patience.

CONTENTS

Introduction 13
Chapter I 17
Chapter II 20
Chapter III 24
Chapter IV 31
Chapter V 34
Chapter VI 42
Chapter VII 48
Chapter VIII 52
Chapter IX 59
Chapter X 64
Chapter XI 67
Chapter XII 71
Chapter XIII 75
Chapter XIV 79
Chapter XV 83
Chapter XVI 93
Chapter XVII 98
Chapter XVIII 103
Chapter XIX 109
Chapter XX 115
Recipes 133
Epilogue 152

INTRODUCTION

Dear Readers:

Overweight is most commonly defined in terms of excess pounds. Physically this is true. Overweight is an illness afflicting the body, but there is a great tendency to forget that what affects the body also affects the mind.

Every overweight person has a different reason for being overweight. What must be realized is that there are no miracle diets, no instant cures, no pills to solve the problem quickly and easily forever. The tendency toward obesity for a person with a weight problem is *always* present; it can, however, be controlled. To this theory we have devoted our book.

This book is a companion to all diets. It can be applied to any diet prescribed by a doctor. It stresses the complete rehabilitation of the person involved, physically and emotionally. We will be covering the long-range aspects of rehabilitation and dealing with the problems occurring before, during, and after weight loss.

Have you ever looked at a pretty object or a lovely scene over and over, day after day, yet suddenly your interpretation of that object or scene took on a fuller, more beautiful meaning? This, in a small way, describes our new outlook on life. Let us share with you our fabulous experience of rebirth.

We don't mean that all of our problems are solved, but because we have a healthier, happier feeling about ourselves, our ability to face these problems as they present themselves is greater. Because we are no longer bogged down with our own emotional and physical inadequacies, we are able to experience more fully the rewards that life presents, and cope more efficiently with the difficulties.

Our compensation has been tremendous. You too can experience this rejuvenation, this fulfillment, this rebirth. Let us share with you our experience of dieting and rehabilitation from beginning to the maintenance of our goal weight. We do not say from beginning to end, for there is no end. An alcoholic is always an alcoholic. A person who has conquered this problem is simply not a practicing one. So it is with obesity. We will always be obese. We have, however, discovered how much food our body needs each day to maintain our goal weight, and how to control our eating habits. So can you.

Perhaps you can identify with one of us as we were many months ago. We each had hit our individual rock bottom. We had one foot in the grave and the other on a banana peel and our loved ones and friends knew it. At this point we both awakened to the realization that our dislike for ourselves and our embarrassment made us ashamed to be seen even by close associates. We did not have a healthy outlook on life and had retreated into a world of unreality. We hope that your weight problem is not as great as ours. But if it is, take heart . . . we have been there . . . we know. . . .

Jean, forty-one, wife, mother of two, and a secretary, traveled down Obesity Lane for many years, and unfortunately took a long time to realize that she was merely existing. Her world began at 6:30 each morning, continued with breakfast, the drive to work, the punching of a time clock at 8:00 A.M. and 5:00 P.M., the drive home, supper, television, and bed. Weekends consisted of housecleaning, washing, ironing, grocery shopping, cooking, and attending church Sunday morning. Her daughter was away at college and her husband's work kept him away from home several nights a week.

This was her life, week after week, month after month. Slipping into something comfortable after work, she began to enjoy her evening solitude more and more, immersing herself in the fictitious existence of television programs and paperback heroines. She pretended to be away when the doorbell rang. The refrigerator provided solace for idle moments.

She began to seriously question her existence when her brother, Jerry, spent the night in town because of a business meeting.

"Why didn't you attend the banquet with Tom last night?" he asked.

"I wasn't invited."

"Are you going to the convention with him next month?"

"No, I have a job, you know."

"That's not the reason, and you know it. I wouldn't take you to a dog fight the way you look now. What are you getting out of life? Better yet, what are you contributing? Why are you living?"

Stunned, words would not come—only tears, and with the tears, release. Holding her in his arms, he quietly told her that she needed to make a thorough evaluation of herself.

Jean began her evaluation by comparing her life to Jerry and Sue's full, happy one; their social life was well balanced with his work load, whereas Jean had no social life. She listened to conversations at the office: fellow staff members discussing shopping excursions, vacation plans, and dinner invitations. She felt unable to enter into any of these conversations. Stores did not stock her large dress size so she made her own clothes. She hadn't planned a vacation in years and was unable to walk even short distances without resting, never dreaming of buying a bathing suit. And, of course, Tom hadn't suggested a vacation either. By comparing herself with others objectively, Jean realized that Jerry was right. Her life had no aim, no direction, little purpose or meaning.

Em's life had no direction either. At age nineteen, she, a college student, knew that it wasn't just baby fat and that she wouldn't grow out of it. She became disinterested and discouraged with the career possibilities she pursued and, having no confidence in herself, she sought other's approval, becoming the image they molded. Away from everyone, she unveiled her true self: depressed, hurt, lonely, and unstable. She bought half gallons of rum and offered drinks to fellow students, drowning her own sorrows and supporting the happy mask she wore as well.

15

Em had never dated and so planned to be away for dance weekends. She wasn't included in trips downtown for dinner or drinks, so she withdrew deeper into her shell and lessened her trust in mankind.

Shortly after she and her closest friend started rooming together, Em became jealous and irritable; Angie had a beautiful figure and a closet full of clothes to match. Em wore one of two pairs of pants and one of three shirts. Angie's comments to others about Em's shabby appearance often drifted back to her. Finally, waking up in the middle of the night in tears scared Em, and she sought the aid of a college counselor.

Yes, each of us had hit our own rock bottom. After years of obesity, traveling thousands of pounds up and down the scale, we knew that we needed a diet—not a fad diet for a couple of weeks, but a diet we could live with for the rest of our lives.

Through friends we learned of an obesity clinic that teaches mental rehabilitation as well as the correct procedure to lose weight. Fortunately we both were able to obtain the financial backing to benefit from this program, and so we began not only our weight loss, but also our beautiful, warm, rewarding friendship. As we learned from the clinic, we drew strength from each other. And through this counseling, care, and concern for one another, we have reached our goal: Jean has lost 100 pounds and Em, 60.

We are so thrilled with these accomplishments that we have written down our experience step by step as we lived them in the hope that we may share with you our good fortune. Won't you accept our hand of helpfulness, encouragement, and friendship, so that you too might benefit from our learning as we have? You *can* lose weight. Join us as we guide you back down the road to a healthier, happier, more beautiful you.

Em and Jean

CHAPTER I

Once begun
A task is easy; half the work is done.
HORACE

Em and Jean each found the same diet clinic right for both of them. Their first few days consisted of apartment hunting, specimen bottles, needles, X-rays, endless blood samples, consultations, electrocardiograms, glucose tolerance tests, and miles of questions about their feelings and attitudes along with their medical histories and medical histories of their ancestors as well. They emerged completely defenseless.

Oh, those photographs! It had been years since Jean had agreed to have her picture taken, yet suddenly she heard a click, and "Now, side view, please." This wasn't the worst.

"Why the pictures?" she asked.

"You'll laugh at them later," was the answer.

"I don't think I could ever laugh at the way I look now."

The physical examinations were next. Jean had not been in a doctor's office, much less on an examining table, for seven years. But there she lay, clothed in nothing but humility. Then came the appointments with the clinic doctors. Em's health was graded A-1; obesity fortunately had not yet taken its toll. Jean's lab tests, however, pointed to hypertension (high blood pressure) and arteriosclerosis (thickening and hardening of the arteries). Did her years of obesity cause these medical problems? Contemplating her hands full of prescriptions and drug bills, she was astounded when told that her weight loss should correct all of her medical complications.

Relieved, they were shuttled to their consultation with the coordinating director of the clinic. Smiling to put Em at ease, he asked how long she had been overweight. After a few quick calculations, she answered, "about twelve years." Smiling again, he startled her: had she walked two miles a day since age fourteen, she might not be in his office today. To Jean's reply of twenty-five years to the same question, his comment was that had she walked a brisk two miles a day from the time of her marriage, she would have no weight problem today. Speechless, her thoughts raced back through her very passive life and the sickening realization of what her inactivity had caused. Gently he brought her thoughts back to the present by describing the program. Along with a diet would be interwoven guidelines for exercise and behavioral therapy. A whole new learning process was about to unfold.

Their final consultations were with the behavioral program director. Em thought his questioning her enrollment on the program must be a joke, for surely the reason was obvious. Why else would anyone go on a diet? Looking at her feet and shifting nervously in her chair, she told him, "I've come here to lose weight . . . ," praying that she wasn't supposed to have any other reason. His prodding of her life at home and college made her realize that obesity was not her only problem. "I've had a few difficulties," she admitted but refused to go into them. She didn't want to take up his time. With a few short comments about the program, and a few papers to sign, that was that.

Because Jean had to delay her start on the dietary program and had begun to analyze the problems causing her obesity, the interview with the behavioral director was short and to the point. After studying her miles of answers, he gave her one of the keys to a new life with one statement: she must

18

learn to get out and be with people more often. Then they were off and running—to the dining room.

* * *

It *is* very important to consult your own physician before beginning any dietary program. Your doctor will prescribe a diet that is right for your bodily needs. Each one of us is physically and emotionally different. That is why it was necessary for us to go through such thorough examinations. Jean's needs were not Em's. A doctor's appointment must be Number One on your list to healthful dieting.

May we also suggest having a friend or photographer take your picture—front and side view. Probably, as we wanted to, you are saying, "I'll bypass the photographs." But don't! Your before pictures will offer encouragement, and yes, believe us, the day *will* come when you will be able to laugh at them. We can remember hiding ours for the first few weeks because of our embarrassment, but no longer. Those pictures are now our reminder of what we once were, and what we could become again if we let ourselves go. But we're getting ahead of ourselves; we will touch on this later.

So, right now you have two things to do:

1. Make a doctor's appointment, and
2. Have your picture taken.

CHAPTER II

Talk of joy: there may be things better
than beef stew and baked potatoes
and home-made bread —
there may be.
DAVID GRAYSON

Complicated directions from a secretary led Em, her father, and Jean and her husband to the dining room. Downstairs, straight ahead, fully uniformed with utensils poised, two smiling women stood behind a cafeteria buffet line. The hungry four rushed to warmers filled with vegetables and vegetable soup and coolers with cottage cheese, salad, peaches, and tuna fish. They were, unfortunately, not allowed some of everything.

The meagerness of their portions was forgotten when they entered the dining room: orange-red carpet, white walls, multi-colored drapes blending beautifully, white pillars parading down the center of the room, white plastic tablecloths, and what seemed like thousands of red signs with bold white letters hung at eye level, placed at each table, plastered on the walls, and in virtually every nook and cranny imaginable. They made sense of none except the NO SMOKING sign.

Many old-timers were eager to explain the program. Jean and Em's first questions, naturally, were about the signs. One in particular really looked ridiculous: ONE MINUTE, TWENTY MINUTES, UTENSILS DOWN, SLOW DOWN. NO SMOKING BEYOND THIS POINT read two signs on opposite sides of the same pillar. Three people sat nearby puffing away unconcernedly. Amazingly enough, explanations made each sign meaningful. "The big signs tell us how to eat. ONE MINUTE means to wait one minute from the time we sit down until we start eating." This was the first rule Jean and Em broke. "TWENTY MINUTES means to make each meal last twenty minutes." This was the second rule broken. Understanding how to make one and a half cups of soup with a few pieces of meat in it last twenty minutes escaped Jean. The rest of the sign, however, explained how: "SLOW DOWN and UTENSILS DOWN mean to stop gobbling and to put utensils down between bites." Jean, unfortunately, was ready for the main course five minutes after beginning her meal.

Em took the special lunch option—a vegetable plate of broccoli, squash, and beets. Eating half of the broccoli, she could go no further. So overwhelmed by the impressive surroundings and nervous about what other surprises were in store, she was unable to force down another bite. Looking anxiously about, Em spotted the meal hours posted in red and white on the wall. She nudged Jean, "Wow! Dinner's at 4:30! And we won't be able to sleep in tomorrow. Breakfast's at 7:30. We made this meal by the skin of our teeth—it starts at 11:30 and ends at 12:30!"

Luckily they had no time to think about growling stomachs. The afternoon was fruitfully spent getting their bearings, searching out accommodations, buying up a storm to outfit their new quarters, unpacking bursting suitcases consisting of every size, shape, and style garb imaginable; quite soon they discovered it was 4:30. This meal, however, their traveling companions gracefully declined, opting to go out and eat somewhere later.

Back in the cafeteria line the two new dieters asked for

everything allowable, and their eyes grew wide at the amount: three separate dishes of aromatic foods, each full, barely leaving enough room on the trays for the lemonade, iced tea, or coffee they were allowed. Their stomachs rumbled with delight at the thought of the roast beef dinner before them, and once again the red and white commandments went unheeded. They did, however, obey the NO SMOKING sign—neither smoked!

Having eaten a few bites in almost animalistic fashion, they settled down and took notice of those around them. Some were eating fish or chicken instead of roast beef, but neither Jean nor Em had seen options in the line. Fish or chicken could be substituted for the meat any night, they learned. Why would anyone want a substitute for roast beef?

With dinner finished and stomachs amazingly full, Em and Jean left to watch their companions eat their supper. Em's father wanted a steak, so the two of them went to a posh steakhouse. Em's only sustenance was water throughout the meal, and her father's succulent sixteen-ouncer didn't even bother her. When he ordered rum cake a la mode piled high with whipped cream and nuts he asked, "Em, my darling, a little bite won't hurt you, will it?" The look on her face conveyed to him that he alone must eat everything put before him.

Tom was leaving the next morning and saw Jean's tears begin to fall. He too had compassion and offered a bite of his cheeseburger. Her hunger, however, was not for food, but for his companionship.

* * *

We found that the sign that gave us the biggest problem and yet was the most important was the sign that read "ONE MINUTE, TWENTY MINUTES, UTENSILS DOWN, SLOW DOWN." Probably, like us, the tendency to gobble your food began from the time you first sat at the table. Admittedly, this presented problems when we were back in our home environment. We were, however, able to conquer our desire to gobble by several techniques. One, television is turned off at mealtime and substituted with relaxing soft music when possible. Second, conversation is a must and, along with it, so is the remembrance to put utensils down as

22

we talk. Third, serving each course of the meal on small individual plates makes the food look not only more appetizing but also larger, making us feel more satisfied with the food we eat at each meal. And after each course, we clear the table of unwanted dishes. Never hurry—strive for a warm, relaxed atmosphere.

Another important point in successful dieting is setting up a regular mealtime schedule and adhering to these times daily. This also discourages the urge to grab a bite (usually the wrong kind) on the run. You may eat your last meal at 5:00 P.M. or at 8:00 P.M.; the time itself is of no moment. What is important, however, is your day to day consistency. If you normally eat at 5:00 and you find you must prolong this until 7:00, look out! Your tendency will be to gobble down everything plus the kitchen sink in ten minutes or less. Ways to help you during this time are discussed later. So set your mealtimes around your own family needs, and, as closely as possible, make this a daily routine.

CHAPTER III

Those who are fond of setting things to
rights, have no great objection to
seeing them wrong.
WILLIAM HAZLITT

Away from the security of loved ones and home, respon-
sible only for rehabilitating themselves, Jean and Em soon
found the days would not be spent in leisure. Drowsily they
fell into the long breakfast line. Approaching their new uniformed friends at what seemed a snail's pace, they peered
into the void warmers and coolers. After showing weekly
meal tickets, they were asked what they would like to eat.

"What can we have?"

Smiling, our friend answered, "You can have six egg
whites, three egg whites and cottage cheese, cottage cheese
and peaches, or one of these dry cereals," as she pointed
behind her. "These are your choices every morning. Today
we also have oatmeal."

Egg whites? What are egg whites? Someone behind them broke into their thoughts and said, "Try the egg whites. Pure protein. Supposedly you lose best eating them . . . gives you more energy to do your walking. They'll cook them with chives if you prefer." Ordering the egg whites answered the question of the slow moving line—each egg white was fried separately when ordered.

"Don't forget your vitamin," they were reminded. Picking up the small white pill cup with a vitamin inside, egg whites, and beverage, they headed for the red and white sea of faces.

Utensils poised, they were caught in the nick of time; they had forgotten to weigh in. Calmly and slowly, those with whom they were eating explained the procedure for filling out the folders they had been given. At the top, each wrote her name, arrival date, expected departure date, initial weight, and goal weight. The rest of the form meant nothing to the new dieters until an old-timer explained. Down one side of the sheet were many headings with twenty-eight columns of boxes representing the days of the month. After weigh-in they entered their weight under the date. The next column represented the daily weight change, controlled by weighing on the same scale before breakfast in approximately the same weight clothing every morning. The next column represented total weight change or the number of pounds lost or gained since the day they had entered the program. Much to their surprise, they had lost a great deal since the previous day: Jean, three pounds, and Em, one. That was initial water weight loss, someone quickly explained, since they were eating much less salt.

The nurse recorded their blood pressure and pulse. Another column was for recording the number of miles walked the previous day. Many dieters offered to show Jean and Em some of their favorite walks. Another column was to record other activities they had engaged in such as swimming, tennis, jogging, exercise class, bowling, and the like. Jean contemplated joining a health spa but Em decided to stick with walking for the time being.

The next column was to record any eating off the program. "Confess!" the row seemed to say. If you were bad yesterday, confess. The two newcomers shuddered at the thought,

"Never!" Their new friends merely smiled and knowingly shook their heads, "We all said that, but it can happen."

The next three boxes would be checked if they had eaten breakfast, lunch, and dinner respectively in the dining room. Their feelings were registered on a scale of one to ten: ten if they were on top of the world, and one if they had jumped off the Empire State Building and were on their way down. Zero was to be entered when ground was reached.

Finishing the charts as best they could, they tackled the now-cold egg whites. "Ugh," Jean commented, and Em heartily agreed. She watched another dieter make egg white crepes and followed suit, sprinkling each egg white with artificial sweetener and cinnamon and rolling it up. Someone else had only three egg whites and added a small amount of cottage cheese to the crepes. To each his own—they had to go down.

At 8:00 A.M. the doctors sauntered into the dining room and sat behind their respective desks while lines formed for folder inspection, question answering, and problem solving. Em was assured her blood pressure and pulse were within normal range and received an A+ on filling out her chart.

Finishing her last drop of coffee, Em took her tray to the clean-up cart and joined some new-found friends for a two-miler.

"Shall we walk through the garden this morning?" one dieter asked.

"Let's do, it's so much prettier," another ventured.

Off they went, leaving Em in a cloud of dust. Thanks to college walking she was able to quicken her stride and catch up. "Come on, Em," one called. "A brisk walk will get your blood circulating. It's time for your body to wake up."

Walk briskly they did, and were soon passing through a beautiful garden that nearly took Em's breath away. Pansies, like splashes of each color of the rainbow, beautifully landscaped, were sprinkled down each side of the walk, paving the way to even more beautifully planned and coordinated settings. An arbored terrace, ladened with wisteria-like ribbons winding around and through the posts, overlooked the scene.

Terraces in long shallow arches paved in gray slate and

engraved with tulip beds of orange, red, yellow, and white led down to the pond—the home of schools of shimmering goldfish. Hills of dogwoods, redbuds, magnolias, and chinese plums complemented the well-manicured lawn. Who could walk briskly surrounded by such beauty? Nonetheless, they forged on.

Stares from passersby which seemed to say "there goes another fatty" escorted the group on their walk. Rounding a corner they approached two pillars with a fence suspended between them—the one-mile marker. Em's companions appeared to have gone crazy patting, kicking, and bowing to the gate posts. "Hi there, Mr. Pineapplehead," one said. Em's staring brought giggles and a point to the top of the pillar. There, majestically perched on the top of the pillars, were large white stone pineapples, the sign of welcome. "Hello, Pineapplehead," Em managed through her laughter, and they all headed back to the dining room for their second mile.

Jean had to delay her first walk to buy appropriate shoes. Golf socks were a must also, she was told, to ward off blisters. Armed with new footwear, she set out alone for "the wailing wall," a four-foot high stone wall having a two-mile circumference, situated only three blocks from her rooming house. She realized her walking would be slower than most, as her previous walking consisted of the distance between the parking lot and her office plus once a week shopping.

"You should be back home in about thirty-five minutes," her friends told her as she prepared for the two-mile journey. Confident she could hold out for an hour, she bravely and briskly began her jaunt. Reaching the wall she found dirt, clutter, no sidewalk, and herself out of breath. Pausing long enough to regain her stamina, she then headed down the gravel path leading around the wall. "Hi, fatty," some people yelled from a passing car. Feeling conspicuous and embarrassed, she rationalized they were just young kids, and studied the beer cans rather than the surroundings as she strode onward.

Turning the second corner of the square after what seemed like hours, she found herself walking on a sidewalk. This side provided easier walking, although it too was cluttered with broken glass, dirt, trash, and piles of fallen leaves. Dodging the cans and ignoring the mocking whistles, she admired the buildings and landscaping inside the wall. Taking her mind off her huffing and puffing by inspecting her surroundings, the last corner seemed to appear much sooner. One more side, then home. This stretch, however, had a small uphill climb and her brisk walk slowed to one-quarter speed. Much weight must be lost before she would be able to really tackle these hills. She arrived home exhausted, but proud of her accomplishment. The walk had taken just under fifty minutes, and she was grateful for the hour she had to rest before dinner.

Apart from walking at least two miles a day, Jean and Em were told that exercise of different sorts was a good way to tone up the loose flab. Some joined health clubs and spas or worked out in gymnasiums if they were unable to walk. The strict regimen of an exercise class helped others.

Jean's rooming friend, Betty, had joined a spa for extra workouts and suggested that she follow suit. She went as Betty's guest one evening after supper but was able to do only a few of the exercises, resulting in a mass of sore muscles the next morning. She resorted to walking for the time being; golf socks had warded off blisters, at least.

With common sense as her guide, Jean planned to walk after breakfast and again after lunch, relaxing, feet up, in between. The third day she had built up to a proud four miles and was able to cope with her schedule. A steaming hot bath after supper brought relief to her cramped muscles so that she could keep on her toes and stick to her structured regimen every day.

One day, Em and Jean were walking around the wall with another friend, Rita, well known for her excessive mileage.

"How many miles have you walked today, Rita?" Em asked.

"Oh, I average about thirteen to sixteen miles a day."

"I'll never walk that much," Jean commented, beginning to feel sore on her fifth mile of the day.

"I don't want to do more than six or seven miles," Em remarked, "because I know that I won't have time to do more than that at home. If I don't keep up my present mileage though, all my muscles will turn to flab."

"Walking is different than most exercises," Rita replied.

"I'm going to decrease my walking gradually about one or two weeks before I leave here. The doctors told me that as long as I walk at least two miles a day at home, no matter how many I have been walking here, I won't get flabby. I figure the faster I get it off, the sooner I'll be going home, looking and feeling great again."

"I always understood that the faster you lose, the more tendency you have of gaining it all back, though. That's why I want to take it off slowly," Em told her, remembering she'd lost only one-quarter pound that morning.

"Anyone can find an excuse not to walk if they really want to, Em. You can find the most amazing rumors in that cafeteria about what is and isn't good for you, and what works best, if you listen hard enough. The doctors have denied that one, though, several times," Rita informed them.

"I've heard stories about sitting in different positions to burn up fat in different places," laughed Jean.

"The only way to find out what's true and what isn't is to ask one of the doctors, I guess, and to experience it yourself," Em commented. They did, and two weeks later Jean and Em were walking between ten and sixteen miles every day.

* * *

Yes, we do urge that you keep a daily schedule. You have heard that figures don't lie. Keeping a chart takes no more than two minutes each day and will pinpoint your errors and emphasize your long suits. Simply get a large ruled notebook and pattern it after ours: date, weigh-in, weight change (loss or gain), miles walked, minutes of activities, eating off your established diet. We caution you to be truthful here. As you will be shown later, you may have established routines that can be rearranged to help you adhere to your diet. And do register your feelings. We all have good and bad days. All of this will be helpful later in analyzing your emotions and dieting achievements.

May we also emphasize that daily physical activity is most important. Brisk walking is one of the best physical exercises a person can engage in, for it touches every muscle in your body. Walk around the block, back and forth several times in a nearby shopping mall on cold rainy days, hike with friends on a beautiful sunny afternoon, and lap up the sun as you stretch your legs at the beach.

We do caution you to begin in moderation as Jean did, with appropriate shoes and, if possible, arms free of cumbersome packages and/or purse. Begin with a mile or two for the first few days. A good measurement is twenty to twenty-five minutes of average walking equals a mile and fifteen to twenty minutes for brisker walking. If you work or perhaps are a student as we are, a twenty minute "brisker" after lunch will be stimulating and rejuvenating as you face the remaining hours of the day. Set up a pattern you can adhere to daily and you will be amazed at the change. We do stress that any question you may have that we do not answer, consult your doctor. Other people can unknowingly lead you astray. Remember, your physician knows you better than anyone.

CHAPTER IV

Just as eating against one's will is injurious to health, so study without a liking for it spoils the memory, and it retains nothing it takes in.

LEONARDO DA VINCI

After four days on the program, the two dieters had established a regular schedule of diet and exercise. Determination to lose the unwanted pounds spurred them on and weight was slowly but surely dropping off. Their only worries were of sore muscles and arriving at the dining room on time. Responsibilities of home and world affairs were far removed.

Reaching the dining room on Thursday morning, they saw a notice on the blackboard: LECTURE 9:00 A.M. —Hypertension. Jean was especially interested, as this was one of her medical problems. Most people are unaware they have hypertension, they were told, and the importance of frequent medical checkups provided by this program was stressed.

Once there is a tendency toward high blood pressure, there will always be that tendency, and it must be controlled. Eliminating salt, its prime cause, is a sure way of its reduction. The group was also cautioned against water-softeners which use salt. With diet and daily exercise, most drugs are unnecessary, they learned. Some of the causes of hypertension were named: chronic kidney disease, hardening of the arteries, and stress. High blood pressure can, in turn, destroy kidneys, cause strokes, blindness, and eventually heart failure.

With a gleam in his eyes and a finger pointing at each one in the room, the lecturer launched his main attack: no one with high blood pressure can overwalk. This brought grins to all faces, since walking was one of his pet remedies. By walking and maintaining diet and exercise, the pounds will drop. One pound of fat burned up by walking creates one pound of water which is then excreted. If the water is not passed right away, there is a temporary weight gain or plateau, but the water will eventually be excreted, and weight loss will follow.

Someone asked, "In order to get rid of the water, do you recommend a diuretic?" The lecturer replied that diuretics show a false weight loss; when they are discontinued, the weight loss also stops until the body has resumed its normal functions without artificial assistance. He assured them that the person who does not take a diuretic will lose the same amount of weight over a thirty day period as the person who does.

* * *

This small chapter, you will find, is one of the most important. There will be times in your dieting when you will experience a weight gain. Prepare yourself now. Every person adjusts differently to dieting. A good rule to follow is that if you *have* strictly adhered to your diet and have a small weight gain, you can deduce the following:

1. You are losing inches, and/or
2. Your body is momentarily holding water. This can also be caused by outside pressure and tension. For some, this loss may take *several days*.

Unless you understand this and prepare for it now, discouragement can counteract all accomplishments you have thus far gained. Chapter X tells how Jean overcame this. If, after a week goes by, you still have not experienced a weight loss, consult your doctor as Jean did. You may be one of us who require less calories per day than most. The sooner you discover this, the better. This can be a very crucial point in your dieting program. So be prepared!

CHAPTER V

Freedom to learn is the first necessity of
guaranteeing that man himself shall
be self-reliant enough to be free.
FRANKLIN D. ROOSEVELT

Introduction to behavioral therapy groups began the first
Friday after breakfast. Jean and Em joined other new pa-
tients in a circle. Each of them was asked his or her reason
for joining the program and their answers were much the
same: to lose weight—30 pounds, 100 pounds, and so on.
Asked how weight loss was intended, their answers were
through diet and exercise.

The therapist explained that the program involved more
than just diet and exercise: their first and main concern was
to be for themselves. They would be changing many old
habits for new ones to include eating patterns, social behavior, keeping the day packed with activities by planning their
time carefully, changing relationships with family and
friends—thereby substituting a new approach to a new life-

style. This would not be accomplished overnight since new habits are not developed quickly and easily. In-depth discussions of habits would be held each week in the groups, taking each topic separately. Overweight people have similar habits and problems and confidentially discussing them within the group would help bring them into better focus for all.

The first habit discussed involved the little black book they had been given. The behavioral therapist explained that these diaries would be effective tools in understanding and correcting problems. Kept accurately, they would provide a record of daily food consumption, weight, and emotional problems vital for changing old behaviors and forming better habits.

Any problem or crisis must be written down: Who were they with? Where were they? What time was it? What happened? Reviewing these notes and discussing them later would help pinpoint the cause and help solve the problem.

Furthermore, the diaries will help determine a weight loss pattern in three to four weeks, showing how much and how fast the patient loses. It is important to forget ultimate goals and to concentrate on weekly weight loss. By losing two pounds a week, the projected goal will be eight pounds in four weeks. When attained, a feeling of self-satisfaction and more determination to work for the next goal will be felt. If, however, this is not enough motivation to set another small goal, a predetermined reward such as clothes, jewelry, books, additions to a hobby—anything other than food—can be set for each accomplishment.

Food and exercise goals for short-term periods should also be set. Having walked two miles yesterday without exhaustion, three miles should be tried today. If this is accomplished, pleasure and more motivation will follow. Successfully structuring one meal at a time will strengthen determination and the scale will bring reward each morning.

One of the most important factors of short-term weight loss, food, and exercise goals is the self-rewarding result. A goal easily reached will be successful. Motivation is the prime factor of dieting. Depression and loss of motivation can cause unstructured eating if the goal is not attained.

The session ended with questions. One newcomer asked

about the red and white signs. The therapist explained that eating is actually a very complex behavior, composed of many small habits. Changing one small habit to more beneficial behavior is encouragement for changing another, and then another, and so on. The red sign stating ONE MINUTE, TWENTY MINUTES, UTENSILS DOWN, SLOW DOWN is a formula for breaking present eating habits. By waiting one minute before eating, becoming accustomed to the presence of food, the habit of digging in and not allowing time to taste and savor each bite can be broken. Utensils should be laid down on the plate after each bite, providing time to enjoy the meal and engage in conversation. Making each meal last twenty minutes gives the body time to begin utilizing the food and become full.

Session over, Em and Jean started out for Pineapplehead.

"Did I understand him right?" Jean exclaimed once they had left the dining room. "I'm supposed to think only of myself here? All my life I've been taught to think of others, and my reward would follow."

Em concurred, "I'm always willing to do something for anyone if they need my help. How could I expect to have anyone come to my aid if I never went to theirs? I was always taught to 'do unto others as you would have them do unto you' and I've always believed in it. Mother always told me that I could expect to get no more out of life than I was willing to put into it."

They walked on for a while in silence, contemplating what the therapist had meant by all of this.

"Actually, I haven't gotten back from others what I have given them a great deal of the time," remarked Em. "I remember just this past semester, a friend of mine was having problems with her boyfriend. She always came to me to talk about things since I knew them both well. Sometimes she asked to talk to me at the most inopportune moments—when I had an exam to study for, when I had plans, or even in the middle of the night. But I always listened and tried to help as best I could, putting all other things aside.

"Then one day I had a problem myself and I thought of her. Surely she'd want to help me, even if only by listening. So I asked her if she could spare a few minutes. She was with her boyfriend and asked if it couldn't wait until the next day;

36

they had planned to go out. I no longer asked for her help, but I was still there whenever she needed me, hoping that someday she would understand that other people had problems too. I never had the heart to turn her down since I didn't want to hurt her as much as she had hurt me."

"My job took its toll on me, too," Jean put in. "I never stood up for myself while blame was put on me for mistakes others had made. I even reached the point of doubting my own ability. Deep down, I know I'm a good secretary, but when others didn't face and admit their own faults, my frustrations grew by leaps and bounds. Basically, I'm a very peaceful person and, like you, could not hurt others as they were hurting me."

"Yes, and I never told my friends I couldn't help them because I was afraid of losing their friendship. I have few enough as it is."

Jean answered, "Then I suppose what the doctor means is that we'll just have to start saying no to some requests. We'll have to think about what we want to do first. Our primary goal is to lose weight, and we can't let anyone or anything hinder our progress."

"This morning someone cut into line for breakfast ahead of me," Em remembered. "Then she even left the line for a cup of coffee in the dining room and came back demanding her egg whites. I know that wasn't right, and it irritated me, but I didn't say anything to her. I guess I should have spoken to her, but I didn't want to create friction. Dieting is hard enough, but if you are on someone's blacklist, and in such close contact with them as we all are, it could become intolerable."

"But, Em, don't you think the people behind you would have appreciated it if you had spoken up? More than one person was behind you in the line, too."

"That's true! It might also help the lady see that she was in the wrong. Then, if she corrected her behavior, others would respect her more."

"We'll just have to evaluate each situation as it occurs, I guess, to see if we should agree or say no. If we have to deny ourselves something to help someone else, and what we want to do is more important to us, we should say no," Em commented thoughtfully. "For instance, my friend at college wanted to talk to me while I was studying for my midterm exams. I should have told her I had an exam the next morning, but I didn't, and consequently my grade suffered. I could understand her saying no to me under the same circumstances. We can't always expect people to be at our beck and call.

"Thinking back, many times when I've said yes against my will or to go along with the crowd, I found myself eating. I eat more when people ask me to do things they could do for themselves. Girls at college sometimes asked me to do their laundry for them on Saturday mornings because I was an early riser and they wanted to sleep in. I did, and it got to the point that they expected me to do it for them every weekend."

"But how do you say no to someone, Em? Do we have to apologize and explain our way out of situations all the time?"

"If we are busy when someone needs us perhaps another time can be offered, or if companionship is needed and we are going out, maybe we could ask them to go with us."

"Well, it's going to take lots of work for me. After forty-one years of living for others, I know I won't be able to change in a day. I'm going to feel pretty guilty for a while."

"Well, at least we can give it a try. If it works, we will be a great deal happier and make other people happier in turn."

"Em, now we have four projects ahead of us," Jean replied with a twinkle in her eyes, "to remember to say no, to write in our diaries, to exercise, and to get to the dining room on time. The only problem I have to write in my diary today is one big sore muscle—all over."

"I'll make a scratch in mine for every time I remember to say no to unreasonable requests. Oh, yes, I must remember to mention the blister on my big toe. Maybe it will turn out to have an effect on my weight loss in the morning."

They laughed, the morning prosperously spent.

While resting that afternoon, Jean's mind kept dwelling on all the things she had learned that morning. Put yourself first, he said. Memories began flooding her mind: buying Tom that sports coat instead of the work shoes she needed badly, buying her daughter the dress instead of dress material for herself, watching the war movie instead of the musical . . . on and on her mind raced. This new concept would take some getting used to, some serious thought, and lots of application.

So began the opening of their pasts, revealing everything: the evaluation—both good and bad, the changing of their ways to make the rest of their lives better than ever before. They knew they were headed in the right direction.

The following Friday they learned the meaning of three new words essential to their behavioral therapy vocabulary: assertive, non-assertive, and aggressive. The assertive person achieves his goals without hurting others, they were taught. The non-assertive person follows other peoples' leadership and keeps his own desires within himself. He often thinks too slowly to respond at the proper time. The aggressive person goes ahead with his own plans regardless of others' feelings.

As several dieters began the morning walk, one newcomer said, "You mean we should say what we want? For instance, last night four of us were discussing going to a movie. Several options were mentioned and, not wanting to rock the boat, I didn't voice my preference. Anything was fine with me."

"That's being non-assertive," another exclaimed. "If you had said what you wanted to see, you would have probably felt much better about it. That shows that honesty and assertiveness must go hand in hand. You weren't entirely honest with everyone since you didn't tell them that you too had a preference."

Jean added, "Well, then, if I were aggressive, I would say, 'Well, it's my car, and I'm going to see the movie downtown, and if you want to come along, you can.' "

Another brought up a college experience. "We found out what the professor wanted and gave it to him whether we thought he was right or wrong, and we were rewarded with an A." Non-assertiveness!

Em's experience was that by going to her professor with her questions, she had a clearer understanding of the subject she questioned, and hence found her assertiveness brought a feeling of individuality and of gaining the respect of her teacher by showing interest in the subject.

Walking along, they heard another in the group, farther back, talking: "There's a woman in the dining room who has been inventing ugly rumors about some of the others on the program and spreading them around to draw attention to herself. I was fed up with her this morning, and I told her I didn't want her sitting at the same table with me. She hurt me by many of the stories, so I hurt her deliberately to pay her back. Good case of aggression, huh?"

"Sounds like you were both pretty aggressive," another exclaimed.

"That's my main problem," the first continued. "I have a mean temper, and although it takes a great deal to make me angry, when I am, I blow my stack and can be very vicious."

Em recalled another experience in which she had been very non-assertive. She was riding to the airport with some friends; one of them had to catch a plane that evening. The driver turned right instead of left at an intersection. "I knew we should have turned left, but said nothing, thinking maybe I was wrong, even though I had been this way once before."

One lady near Em said, "By voicing your opinion you would have spared them a great deal of precious time, I'll bet."

"You're right. We got hopelessly lost, and when we finally found where we were, we had to break the speed limit to get to the airport on time. We arrived one minute before the plane took off."

Learning to be assertive is learning a whole new way of life. Every person in the group had his own story of his past behavior, and each had a great deal to think about, to work on, to change. The therapy would help them, and they were also willing to help themselves.

* * *

As we touched on before with the daily schedule, diaries can be a tremendous help in pinpointing, understanding, and correcting our many problems if kept accurately and honestly. Foremost is the word *honestly*. It is not necessary that you show your diary to anyone else, but it *is* important that you see for yourself what you truly are. And from this point you can begin constructively changing and building.

A little three-by-five notebook can serve this purpose. Each day record your weight, what you ate for each meal, if you were unstructured with your diet, what you ate if you were (and this means *every mouthful*), any emotional problems you encountered, mentioning the time, where you were, and whom you were with. As you analyze these pages later you may observe patterns or habits that can be eliminated or substituted with something more constructive.

Remember, too, rewards are very important. They need not be expensive. Here is one idea that may help. An obese person most always rewards himself or herself with mouthfuls of yummies, right? Why not put that fifty or seventy-five cents you would normally have spent on the yummies into a little bank or small box on your dresser. Then, when you have lost, say, five pounds, you will have funds for a much more valuable reward—a replacement for what could have been more pounds on you.

Another point we would like to bring out is that whatever mold you may find yourself in—aggressive, assertive, or non-assertive—you will find changes that must be made. Your primary concern now is your weight loss. *Your* needs must come first, and this is a very vital key to your success. Begin now by analyzing your own habits so they can be altered to this end. Just adhering to a diet is not enough. Not only your physical, but your mental and emotional being must undergo a step by step change to be a healthier, happier you.

The more open and honest you learn to be with others, the more you will find yourself contributing to conversations, especially at meals, when people relax and take a break from work. By speaking up at mealtime, it is easier to slow down your eating, allowing more time to digest your food which makes you feel full on a smaller amount of food. No matter what the diet, feeling satisfied with the amount of food you are allowed is a crucial factor, and slowing down is the way to accomplish this most effectively.

You can build a better you. Stay with us; we will show you how!

CHAPTER VI

Every man is the architect
of his own fortune.
SALLUST

In the short time they had been on the program, not even two weeks, Jean and Em had become accustomed to their eating and exercise routines, but found little to do at night. Television became monotonous night after night, and the supply of novels was wearing thin. They had to find something to do.

Em was invited to go dancing one night but didn't really want to go. An evening of watching other people dance made her feel lonely and unattractive. She went to the discotheque only because it provided a change in the evening routine and she had heard constant chatter in the dining room about it the previous week. By going, she hoped to be accepted by the in-group. This event, however, proved to be no different than other dances she had attended. Unable to start a conversation, Em sat for four hours feeling sorry for herself. She waited for the people she had come with to make a move to leave; they, however, were having a good time and were unaware of Em's depression. Finally noticing an acquaintance leaving, Em asked for a lift home. She was embarrassed to ask her friend to go out of her way, but was assured the few extra miles were of no consequence. Em decided against that form of evening entertainment for the future. There were, however, many others sources of evening entertainment in the area—movies, shows, and club meetings open to the public. Health spas had evening hours. They had to keep their eyes and ears open.

Em became close friends with the lady who had taken her home from the dance. One night at supper, they decided to see a movie that evening and had a marvelous time. The movie was light and fun and took their minds off dieting and troubles, putting them in another situation for a few hours. Em never forgot that evening with June; it was one of the most enjoyable she spent on the program.

Rainy days were terrible. Boredom, since walking is so unpleasant in the pouring rain, and idleness are devastating to dieters and must be dealt with. Thoughts of food are prominent when the mind is idle. For those days hobbies and projects began working themselves into Jean's and Em's daily structure. Em took up knitting since her sister was to have a baby in August. Sewing, ceramics, plans for remodeling, and many other projects for which they had never before found time kept their minds and hands busy, and were good antidotes for boredom. When tired and hungry, naps were the best solution.

One lady kept herself busy during the day by planning a party for ten guests. She absorbed herself in the preparations, providing something new and different for those invited. Handiwork would keep their fingers busy while conversation would stimulate their minds.

Jean didn't want to go to Ruth's party, but could think of no plausible excuse for not going. She was secure in her day's routine and evenings were spent reading, watching television, writing letters, and going to bed early. Tired from carrying her excess baggage, she needed plenty of rest. Analyzing further, she was not ready to leave the security of her routine for social events, not knowing what would be discussed, nor what would be served. She heard rumors that low calorie candies and diet drinks were to be offered. Also, still rationalizing, she had no clothes suitable other than everyday walking slacks. Betty, her rooming companion, was also invited and persuaded Jean to go, assuring her that she also had no appropriate clothes, but that getting out would do them both good. Betty also pointed out that they might lose friends by not appearing.

They did go, and had a marvelous time. The attire ranged from slacks to hostess gowns, making everyone feel at home. Passing up the diet candy was not hard for Jean. She wasn't really hungry after the big supper that had been served and also was motivated not to eat by the presence of other dieters. The diet drink was her only refreshment. Glancing around the room, she noticed several nibbling on the candy and taking seconds. Later in the evening one of the group played several of her own renditions on the piano, providing a beautiful climax to a lovely evening.

Thanking the hostess, Jean and Betty drove toward home. "Did you notice Toni was unable to leave the candy alone?" Betty commented. "I talked with her about it and she just couldn't stop once she started. It was like sliding down a mountain."

"Was she really hungry?"

"No, you remember the big meal we had tonight, and she ate every bite. But she just couldn't pass up the candy. Did you eat any?"

"No, just the drink. Maybe the answer is never to take the first bite."

"Next time, for added security, we'll sit together and you nudge me if I weaken."

Laughing, Jean agreed, reminding Betty that she might need the nudging. Thanking her for pushing her into her first social event, Jean realized how non-assertive she had been, having attended the party because Betty hadn't wanted to go by herself. She had momentarily forgotten one of the doctor's evaluations of her needs: to get out and be with people more often.

Em was greeted upon arrival at Ruth's party by a small tray of candies and a diet drink. She wasn't prepared to assert herself and say no to temptation, but managed. The doctors had told her that the amount of calories eaten was not as

44

important as breaking the nibbling habit. Looking around, she saw that a few people had eaten their candy, and others were fidgeting nervously, trying to control their desire.

Cameras flashed throughout the party, and Em kept her head constantly bent over her knitting, not wanting her picture taken. Asserting herself, she told everyone how she felt; picture taking made her feel nervous and uncomfortable. The low whispers across the room, undoubtedly about her immature behavior, brought a big lump to her throat, but she was unable to express herself without being aggressive and getting angry or walking out. She felt ugly and didn't want her feeling captured on film. Trying to ignore the circulating comments, she concentrated on helping Ann, with whom she had come, with her knitting. What seemed like fifty rolls of film later, flashcubes stopped popping and she and Ann took their leave. Ann took her candies home to her husband.

Once in the car Ann burst. Em knew that Ann had had a rough time resisting temptation, and realized talking it out would relax them both.

"Em, that was so hard! You know, it may sound strange to you, but I find that some foods hum to get your attention, some beckon you to eat them, and some even yell, 'Hey, look over here! Eat me! Eat me!' Those are the ones I find hardest to resist because I like them the best, like peanut butter and ice cream and cake. I'm glad Ruth put the candies on trays, though, because I find they are much easier to resist than when they're put in my hand. It's strange but it seems as though a string is attached to my hand over which I have no control; if something edible is put into it, it automatically goes into my mouth. One of my friends here, Lee, has a tendency to buy cookies and eat them, bags at a time. When I'm with her she literally puts the cookies in my hand. No matter how wrong I know it is, it goes right to my mouth. She just wants to share her guilt, and I know I should have more control, but I don't."

"Did you put all that in your diary, Ann? Maybe all your trouble occurs with Lee buying the cookies. Maybe you should stay away from her when you know she is going shopping. Or maybe it's just the supermarket you should avoid. Does it happen only at certain times of the day? I'll walk with you at those times if you want me to."

45

"Well, Dr. Therapist . . . ," and both girls broke into peals of laughter.

"Seriously, though, Em, my problem isn't just at the supermarket; I have trouble at home, too. My husband brings home candy—the good kind—and I eat it when he isn't looking. I just don't know what to do."

"Wow! You do have a problem. That would be a great group discussion, Ann. Let's bring it up next session." Saying good night, Em went upstairs, her mind racing about the problems of unstructured eating. "How can I avoid it if I am tempted?" she wondered. "The candies weren't very appetizing tonight, but what if it had been cheesecake, ice cream, or peanut butter?"

Activity and companionship deterred Jean and Em from unstructured eating this time. They teamed up with others each day for walking and spending free time. One of them always thought of something to do when boredom struck. This way the days sped past pleasantly without much chance to think about eating, except at mealtime. Their stomachs became geared to mealtimes, places, and portions; they became hungry when it was time to eat and when they entered the dining room, but seldom at any other time or place. They were in the process of changing their first few habits, and their accomplishments gave them great satisfaction: doing things they hadn't done in a long time, having fun together while doing them, and watching the scale go down steadily as a result—all rewards for their hard work.

* * *

Boredom, loneliness, and tension are the three main pitfalls of successful weight loss. By self-analysis now, you can determine your problem spots, and begin your own treatment. Each day should be planned *ahead of time* including what you will eat, what you will wear, your activities with friends, exercise, a certain amount of time to yourself, a certain amount to rest, and a time to write in your diary. Make your own itinerary. We do caution you, however, that you can plan too tight a day. Too much activity can be just as detrimental as too much idle time. A good book or hobby is an excellent substitute for last minute change of plans. Begin now by creating these new "good" habits. Before long you

46

will be able to pace your activities and your time schedule so that these three pitfalls are eliminated.

May we also caution you to be prepared when attending a party or other social gathering. There is bound to be food abundant there. If possible, find out beforehand to what kind of activity you are invited and what is to be served. As Em discovered, the less surprises, the easier it will be to remain structured. Take some advice from old pros: DON'T TAKE THAT FIRST BITE OF UNSTRUCTURED FOOD! You will find admiration for sticking to your diet far outweighs the gibes.

CHAPTER VII

A fat kitchen, a lean will.
BENJAMIN FRANKLIN

At breakfast the next morning, the problems encountered at Ruth's party were discussed. Beth was anxious to know what had been at the root of her lack of self-control.

"I just don't seem to have any will power. I can't say 'no' even when I should. Isn't there some way I can make myself stop being unstructured? I must be one of those people who just can't diet."

An old timer spoke up. "I have much the same problem, and I still don't have it licked . . . it takes a great deal of work. I have learned, however, there is no such thing as will power. We can't be expected to pass up food when it is shoved under our noses, and we mustn't blame ourselves for being unstructured under those conditions. The doctors say the solution is to control our environment. If we can't resist peanut butter, we should avoid it. We mustn't feel obligated to serve nuts and nibbles at parties just because everyone else does and because we have done so for years. We should serve something we personally don't like, but which others do, or, if there isn't anything we don't like, serve only what we can eat. If we're unstructured, it is much better for our weight if we eat a carrot stick or a cucumber slice instead of bacon dip on a potato chip, or nuts, or cheese and crackers."

"What if we go out somewhere, and are tempted, like last night, though?" insisted Toni.

"Find out what will be served beforehand, and if you feel you won't be able to resist, don't go; or ask your hostess please not to serve you. She will understand, and will respect you for not wanting to break your new habit and for losing weight. We must be assertive when these situations occur."

"What if your husband brings things into the house for himself and, when he isn't looking, you eat them! I have a terrible craving for candy, and my husband always brings it into the apartment. I can't leave it alone," Ann confessed.

"That's where a contract comes in. Obviously the only way you'll stop eating his candy is for him not to bring it home, so ask him not to bring it back to the apartment, but please to eat it elsewhere. If he refuses, you make a contract. You say to your husband, 'I'll diet and lose weight if you will stop bringing candy into the house.' If this doesn't satisfy him, re-evaluate the contract until you both are benefiting equally from it. If you've been stubborn about not letting him buy new golf clubs he really wants, you can offer that as a bargain: golf clubs for him, no candy for you. The contract must be equally beneficial; otherwise one person will resent it. You aren't inferior, and therefore shouldn't feel guilty for standing up for your own rights ... you have as many as he does."

"I remember a time when my father made a contract with me," Em related. "I was sixteen and wanted to get my driver's license. My father said I could, providing I practice shifting gears on the lawnmower. I knew the lawnmower gears weren't actually shifted and could only be moved while the riding mower was stationary. The gears controlled the speed, and nothing else. However, I agreed to mow the lawn, as getting my license was important to me. I have always been taught not to contradict my elders. The deal was unfair and I knew it. I found out later my non-assertiveness only reduced my father's respect for me."

"I have a problem when I walk by a drug store," another old-timer related. "I always have a tendency to stop in and buy penny candy. The therapist suggested that I not bring loose change when I go past the drugstore or when I'm walking. It's been hard to adjust to, but it really has helped. I think the main thing is to stop a situation before it becomes a problem—to anticipate upcoming problems, recognize patterns and situations that commonly lead us to destruction, and solve them before they even become problems."

"When I began the program, my landlady offered me kitchen privileges," recalled Jean, "but I knew that if I were to go into the kitchen with the tempting aroma of good food everywhere, I would be doomed. So I declined and thanked her for the offer, explaining that I lack will power, and I took the room upstairs. I knew I had to stop that situation before it became a problem."

"What do we do if we have an irresistible urge to eat, though?" asked Toni. "I just get plain starved at times, and can't control my urges."

"That has happened to me, too, and I've found that the best thing to do is walk—not necessarily with anyone. Somehow just walking calms my hunger down immensely." Laughing, Em cited an example: "A friend of mine once brought to my attention the fact that cows, when they are being fattened for slaughter, are put in very small quarters and fed, and are never allowed to exercise. The others, however, are allowed to roam the fields, and they are the ones that tend to eat less. It's a funny analogy, but quite true. It's amazing how many obese people have never exercised while those who have no weight problem usually do."

"Being with friends when we are hungry reminds me that I always have more control when I'm with a companion. I feel guilty when I'm unstructured, but at least when I sneak eat no one else will condemn me. I even put my candy wrappers in the trunk of the car and throw them away in a public trash can instead of at home," Betty stated.

"The friend who took me from the discotheque confessed after a movie that had I not been with her, she would have bought some popcorn," Em remembered.

"But at the same time, there are friends with whom you know you can be unstructured. When Lee and I go shopping,

I know she will buy something unstructured and delicious, and persuade me to eat it with her. Sharing her goodies lessens her guilt," Ann volunteered.

"Well, Ann, if Lee causes you to be unstructured, then you shouldn't be with her. Can you make a contract with her that you will walk with her if she doesn't buy any food? That way you'll be doing her a favor by helping her lose weight faster as well as helping yourself."

"You're right, Jean. I know when I'm structured, I lose. Maybe she'll feel better when she sees the scale start to drop, giving her motivation to stay structured more often. It will take some time, though, because the habit is so deeply ingrained now."

It was time to walk and they all grabbed their trays, teamed up with walking friends, and headed for Pineapplehead.

* * *

There is no such thing as will power. How true this is. We *must* CONTROL our environment. And this is just as true for us now after reaching our goal weight as it is for you. We *still* make contracts with our family and friends. As we said in the Introduction, an obese person is always obese. This is why it is so important that good habits are established now: they must remain with you the rest of your life.

To CONTROL your environment, you must be one step ahead all the time. As we stressed before, plan your daily activities ahead; learn to anticipate your and your family's moods and desires and be prepared. If, for some reason, you are unable to cope with a particular situation, back off and analyze the problem. If possible, take a walk. Walking will relieve the tension and give you time to think more clearly. Strive for calmness; CONTROL will follow.

CHAPTER VIII

When you feel how depressingly slowly
you climb,
It's well to remember that
Things Take Time.
PIET HEIN

As Em's fourth week on the program drew to a close, she became increasingly anxious since her mother was arriving next week for a visit. Em still wore the same clothes she had worn when she left home; she had lost twenty pounds since then, but could see no change.

She brought her anxieties to the attention of her fellow dieters during the next group session. She felt awful about taking up everyone's time with her own problems, but soon realized the sessions had been established for this exact purpose. Everyone tried their best to help and made many useful suggestions. She also found that her problems were not unique, and discussing them openly helped many others in the group.

Em introduced her problems by stating she felt her mother would see no change and would be disappointed in her apparently minimal progress. "Then my parents will want to take me home," she told them. "I'll have to tell her how much I've lost and how much I weigh. I've never admitted these things to anyone because I'm embarrassed to discuss them."

"Then don't! Be assertive and tell your mother you don't want to discuss the numbers. Explain that we are being taught here to put less emphasis on the scale and more on ourselves," one of the group suggested.

"But what if they decide that I can't stay unless I prove to them I'm doing a good job?"

"You don't have to name figures for that. She'll be able to see it in you, and also in your attitude change. You don't have to tell them anything you feel is personal if you don't want to."

"But it's their money that's putting me through the program. Don't they have a right to know?"

"Certainly not. If they didn't trust and love you enough to have the confidence that you would complete the job, they wouldn't have spent the money in the first place."

"I've never stood up to my parents before to voice my opinion. I don't know how to be assertive without being aggressive. I don't understand where one stops and the other starts."

The therapist suggested playing roles as a practice for what Em would say to her mother. Em was to be herself and Ann was selected to play the part of her mother.

Em told her "mother" exactly how she felt about talking about weight and diet. Ann made many remarks typical of her mother, which made the role playing valuable. The practice helped her gain poise and self-confidence. They practiced using the guidelines provided by the therapist: Em stopped shifting from one foot to the other and stood firm, not wringing her hands nor looking down at her feet, but straight at Ann; kept her voice at an even pitch, low and soft, without anger, yet firm in tone; looked Ann straight in the eye, kept her face from tensing and did not let her eyes grow bright with anger or reproach, hurt or guilt; countered Ann's every statement with one of her own, without hesitation or using

53

"um," "ah," "er," and "well"; and chose her words carefully to convey her meaning with the correct emphasis, to make her points clear and concise without one "I'm sorry," for she had nothing to be sorry about and everything to be proud of. After practicing with Ann, she became quite proficient and her anxiety decreased greatly.

Another worry Em had about her mother's impending visit was the possibility that she would compare Em's weight loss with that of her sister's on a similar program three years prior. "She's bound to compare us, and I know that I haven't lost as much as she did. I have always been compared to my sister because she is ten years older than I, and we are the only children. I've grown somewhat accustomed to the comparisons, but it still hurts to be constantly reminded of my faults and her assets. Should I call my mother before she comes to warn her that I haven't done as well as my sister?"

"Oh, no, don't apologize! The comparisons are unjust and unfair to you. Let your mother judge your weight loss for herself when she comes. If you really want to call first, talk to her in a positive manner. Tell her you have done your best, that you have stayed structured and done all the right things since you came down here, and that everyone is proud of you. We all *are* proud of you, Em, and we can see how well you've done, and we won't hesitate to let your mother know our feelings."

"That's right!" many others confirmed, which drowned Em's doubts and brought tears to her eyes. For the second time she accepted the love she could not ignore. The first time was when her parents told her she could join the program. Em had many friends here and they conveyed their love 100 percent.

Eating in a restaurant was also discussed as Em would have to face this for the first time next week. The therapist gave some helpful guidelines for eating out: what to eat must be decided before anything else when planning restaurant meals. A restaurant serving foods allowed on the program should be chosen and reservations should coincide with normal meal time.

Eating must be done no differently than in the diet cafeteria: slowly, pausing before starting for one minute, and putting down the silverware between bites, thereby making the meal last twenty minutes. Take the initiative to make conversation, they were instructed. Only when the atmosphere is comfortable will bad habits be easily resisted.

They were told to decide what to order before they entered the restaurant. Once there, dinner companions must understand that excess food on the table was a terrible temptation to the dieter: bread, cheese, and crackers are not allowed and will power is non-existent. The waiter will remove them from the table if asked.

"Oh, I couldn't do that!" one group member exclaimed. "I wouldn't feel right having all the goodies taken away just because I couldn't have them. What if many people are with me? I would think it very selfish to ask that everything be removed for my sake. I'd really feel guilty. No, I don't think that's right at all."

"You're the one with the problem, though," another countered. "They can eat those things whenever they want; one meal doing without won't kill them. If they asked you out to eat, they most probably already know that you are on a diet, and are planning to eat accordingly themselves. They will respect you for doing everything possible not to go off your diet."

"I make a joke out of it when I go out," one businessman recounted. "I just tell them how much money one bite of cheese or bread would cost me. If I gained two pounds from eating it, and my average loss is two pounds a week, I've lost three weeks time: I gained back last week's pounds, plus it will take me another week to lose them, and at the same time I have lost this week's two pounds because I had to spend it losing two more. In other words, instead of losing six pounds, I would have only lost two in the three weeks, and at the amount we spend on this program each week; that is a great deal of money! Everyone thinks it's really funny and we all laugh, but the temptation is removed from the table without hurt feelings, even if I had never previously met the people with whom I am dining."

"I don't have those problems," Em said, relieved. "Food I can't eat doesn't bother me. I'd rather watch others have the enjoyment of eating it. I really wouldn't get any enjoyment out of it myself because I would feel so guilty for having been unstructured. Plus, I couldn't possibly be unstructured with my mother watching!"

The discussion drew to a close and Em felt much more

confident that she could handle her mother and her questions. She called home and practiced her assertiveness by telling her mother that she was losing well, but during her visit not to discuss weight loss. Em could only assure her that she was doing her best. She cautioned her mother against presupposing her appearance and also asked not to be compared with her sister. Her mother understood and, after hanging up, Em was even more sure she would stay in control throughout her mother's visit.

On Tuesday, when her mother arrived at the airport, Em found that all her anxieties had been for naught. Her mother noticed the weight loss immediately. Pleased and proud, she wanted to rush out and buy Em new clothes. Em, however, became assertive and explained that buying new clothes now would be foolish.

"Anything we buy now, I'll have to discard. Remember, Mum, I'm going to need a whole new wardrobe when I reach goal!"

"Yes, I want you to throw out all your old clothes when you are finished. Forget trying to take anything in. Your father and I have worked hard for many years for you and your sister, and we can now afford to buy you a new wardrobe of well-deserved clothes."

Thrilled, Em's fears vanished. She knew, however, one dreaded question was inevitable: "How much do you weigh?" When her mother finally did ask, Em responded with her much rehearsed speech: "I have been losing well and will continue to do my best. My weight now is insignificant, since I won't weigh the same tomorrow, and what I weigh now means nothing to what I will weigh at goal. We have been taught to put less stress on the scale, and more on ourselves and our daily structure."

The poise, smile, and firmness without hostility were perfect. Answering so directly, Em saw her mother at first a bit taken aback, but then came understanding and with it the promise not to ask again. Em had surprised herself as well, and seeing her mother's favorable reaction gave her confidence and erased any guilt feelings. She remained in control and could hardly wait to tell her friends. Em introduced her mother to many dieters and each expressed great pride in Em's progress. When hearing their praise, Em felt embarrassed, and yet proud to have such wonderful friends.

The only problem encountered was eating out with her mother that night at a fancy steakhouse. Em went prepared, her menu planned ahead. Ordering was no problem. Then trouble began. Having discussed with other dieters the problems of restaurant eating, her mother signaled the waitress and asked to have the cheese, bread, salad dressing, olives, pickles, salt, pepper, cream, and sugar removed from the table immediately. Horrified and extremely embarrassed, Em calmly told the waitress not to bother, confusing the waitress no end.

"Mum, the things on the table don't bother me the least bit. I'm looking forward to eating my steak. Don't deny yourself the delicacies just because I'm here. Depriving you would make me uncomfortable. If I want something removed, I'll ask, I promise."

Em's mother listened attentively and did not interrupt, and from then on treated her as she wanted and needed to be treated—as an individual with her own feelings and opinions. This was a major breakthrough.

More problems arose, however, when the main course arrived. Em told her mother beforehand she didn't want to discuss the diet during supper; she wanted to enjoy her meager five-ounce steak and pretend it was a big twenty-four-ouncer, just like everyone else's. Having forgotten the agreement, her mother asked about calorie counts. Em, quite close to becoming aggressive, overcame her rising temper and calmly and firmly changed the subject, talking about home and family instead. The meal was by no means a pleasant one, but Em learned a great deal about assertiveness, its positive effects, and the lack of guilt with it. She learned more about herself, as did her mother.

Em's mother left the next day, respect and pride glowing in her eyes. Em was very pleased with the way everything had turned out and grateful for the relief from the tensions she had been through the past two weeks. Only when she returned to her apartment that evening did she realize how much it all had taken out of her—she slept for fourteen hours solidly.

* * *

As you have learned from Em's experience during her mother's visit, she had to utilize all facets of what she had thus far learned. She discovered that a regimented diet *must* go hand in hand with behavioral therapy if success is to be achieved. Dieting alone will not work; there are too many emotional crises that can throw us off. We must learn to deal with these crises *so our dieting will be successful*. This is why so many dieters fail to achieve goal. They simply cannot cope emotionally.

Each of us has different obstacles to face. Jean's emotional turmoils were of a different nature as you will learn in the next chapter. Whatever your own problems are, the important thing to remember is that all difficulty *can* be resolved by practicing over and over the good habits and therapy you are learning throughout these chapters.

CHAPTER IX

Of all the passions, fear weakens
judgment most.
CARDINAL DE RETZ

Jean's first trip home after four weeks on the program came about because of a summons to appear at a jury trial resulting from her son's death two years prior, caused by a car-train collision. Worrying about the trial and the questions that would be asked, she began to show signs of wear in several ways. The week before departure, her blood pressure began increasing and her weight loss diminished. In fact, one day she even gained weight. Knowing that she had been structured and had walked seven or eight miles each day, Jean tearfully got in line to see the medical director during breakfast.

After she explained the reason for her scheduled trip home, the doctor told her the weight gain was probably due to water retention caused by tension and pressure and asked to see her blood pressure recording each morning. If it became exceedingly high, medication would be necessary.

Jean lost only three-quarters of a pound over the nine-day period before she flew home but, fortunately, had not required medication.

Looking forward to seeing her family again, Jean hoped they would notice her twenty-pound loss. Her clothes were quite loose, but she had decided against buying anything new for the visit since spending money on something she would only be able to wear a few times seemed ridiculous. She packed two old dresses and wore the prettiest one home, fastening the belt several notches tighter than four weeks previous.

Stepping off the plane, Jean's elation was unimaginable as her daughter, Connie, ran out to greet her and her husband tried to hold back tears. After putting the luggage in the car, they drove to the nearest supermarket. "Our cupboards are bare," Connie told her mother. Connie filled the cart with the things she and her father could eat, and Jean, determined to stay structured, selected only those items on her diet.

Jean suggested eating before driving home as it was now her mealtime, and her conditioned hunger alarm clock was ringing. Stopping at a cafeteria, they chose their own meals. Jean had a lettuce salad with vinegar dressing, broiled fish without tartar sauce, and iced tea. Having eaten these in the dining room, she knew they were permissible; she even managed to leave some fish on the plate.

Reaching home, they were greeted by neighbors, all eager to hear about her life on the program. All were amazed at her walking eight miles a day and dieting at the same time. Jean filled them in as best she could about the diet, and they brought her up to date on all the happenings at home.

The next morning they were due at the courthouse at 8:30. Picking the members of the jury would be the first order of business. Around 1:00 P.M. the six jury members were chosen and everyone was dismissed for a forty-five minute lunch break.

Jean's growing anxiety over the trial and the lateness of the lunch hour was almost too much to cope with. She rallied though. Tom, Connie, and a dear friend Virginia helped her stay structured. She ordered the only permissible food on the menu: cottage cheese and peaches. They gobbled the food and rushed back to the courtroom. Their lawyers were there and motioned them to enter. Jean, soon realizing she could not remain in the room and listen once again to the details of her son's death, excused herself and sat on the bench outside for the remainder of the day. After a recess, Connie and Virginia remained outside also. Staying outside the courtroom was almost as nerve-racking as listening to it all.

On the way home Tom described what had been brought out by their lawyers. At home Connie and Jean broiled chicken, threw a vegetable on to boil, and called it supper. No one was hungry. Tom made strong drinks, but Jean managed to decline and substituted a diet drink. "A drink will steady your nerves," Tom insisted, but she remained firm and structured.

The next morning they were back at the courthouse, having had very little sleep. Again, the three stayed outside with the witnesses. Lunch was a repeat of the day before. Tension mounted as time for them to take the stand drew close. Virginia was told she would be called the next day. That night all took sleeping pills to get some much needed rest.

None of them had been called to the stand Wednesday morning and, even though their lawyers assured them things were progressing smoothly, nervousness and apprehension continued to mount. No longer could Jean face the cottage cheese and peaches for lunch. Tom said it was time she ate something decent and ordered the meat loaf special for all. Jean ate about half plus salad with vinegar dressing. Feeling guilty about her first unstructured eating only added more stress. Virginia was called to testify as a character witness just before the judge called a halt to the proceedings for the night. Connie, Tom, and Jean would testify the first thing Thursday morning.

Jean accepted the drink Tom made that night and immediately became ravenously hungry. She wanted to eat everything in sight. Connie knew her mother felt bad about lunch and prepared only the food Jean could eat. Weighing herself Thursday morning, Jean had gained two pounds since leaving the program. She vowed to stay structured that day, no matter what happened.

By the time they finished testifying that morning none felt they could swallow more than coffee; this they drank by the gallons. The personnel behind the lunch counter in the dime store across the street became quickly accustomed to this, and upon seeing one of them coming, immediately began pouring. The testifying was over around 4:00 Thursday afternoon and the wait for the jury's verdict began. They waited and waited. No one dared leave. Finally, around 9:00 P.M. someone counted noses and bought cheeseburgers, french fries, and cokes for everyone. All was devoured in about ten minutes—Jean finished first.

Finally, around midnight, the judge called the jury back into the courtroom to see if they were near a decision. They said yes, but would like to finish tomorrow, as everyone was exhausted. After some discussion, the judge dismissed them until 10:00 A.M. Walking to the car, Jean was aware of swollen ankles and realized the cheeseburger and french fries had been loaded with salt; for the last few weeks, she had been salt-poor on her diet. Arriving home, she found her ankles as large as her calves. She had to carry her shoes into the house.

Getting on the scale the next morning, Jean had gained another five pounds. Her ankles were still not their normal size, but the swelling had gone down considerably, and she was able to squeeze into her shoes.

Back at the courtroom once again, they waited until 3:00 that afternoon, at which time the jury ruled in their favor. Their victory however was to be short-lived. Their lawyers felt sure that the case would be appealed to a higher court. All for nothing, and seven pounds to boot!

They had a barbecued chicken supper that night.

Jean refused even to look at the scale on Saturday morning and decided to fast all that day and Sunday, having planned to fly back to the program Sunday afternoon. While Jean was asleep, Tom, Connie, and Virginia agreed she was not emotionally ready to return to the program. Later, Jean listened to their reasoning and agreed to change the flight to one week later. Virginia suggested that she stay with her the next week; Connie was returning to college and Tom was leaving for a business trip. "I'll even walk with you," she said. So it was arranged that Jean stay with Virginia, providing the opportunity to become structured again and to lose some of the gained weight.

She did not fast, remembering the doctor's warning against

this normal post-binge reaction, and realizing that he was right; her body and mind were not ready for such drastic measures. Virginia and Jean dieted, walked, rested, dieted, and walked some more, Sunday through Saturday. By Sunday morning she had lost the seven pounds gained plus an additional three. Their jubilation increased when, hopping on the scale after Jean, Virginia found she had lost two pounds herself. Everyone was pleased with their accomplishments and Jean could look once again to the future with renewed determination. The rehabilitation program was working.

* * *

The main thrust of Jean's trip home brings out that there are times we will not be able to control our environment; there will be times when problems overpower us and drag us under. When this happens it is best to get with an understanding friend (either personally or by phone) to whom you can unburden yourself. Then slowly talk your way back on your diet. If possible, start walking so clear thinking will come. Next, get right back on your program—the *next* meal. Jean's idea of fasting, hoping to make up for her lost days, is out. Believe us, it does not work. You may be able to fast for a few meals, but when you begin your dieting program again, the tendency is to be unable to stop eating once you begin. You are already in a weakened mental state and the best procedure at such a time is to rely on your newly established habits. As you read, once Jean got back on her daily routine at the next meal her motivation returned. So will yours.

The Reader's Digest Family Word Finder tells us that the origin of the word *diet* comes from the Greek *diaita* which means "course of life." You are learning just that, to change your long-term eating habits and to master a new way of living. Let us guide you through the next phase in the process of rehabilitating your mind and body. Ready?

CHAPTER X

Flops are a part of life's menu, and I've never been a girl to miss out on any of the courses.
ROSALIND RUSSELL

Back on the program once again, Jean was most anxious to weigh in, and was overjoyed to find she had dropped four pounds since her departure two weeks before. All of her friends were happy about her success and welcomed her back. Discussing the eating problems at home with a few close friends, Jean saw they too were appalled at the cheeseburger gain, and were very proud of her restructuring.

She soon settled down into her old established routine. As the days passed, however, her weight loss became almost nil, and along with it her spirit and determination. Although completely structured, the feeling she wasn't accomplishing anything became acute. Group sessions no longer helped reassure her. The urge to binge, to go out and eat everything in sight, charged into her thoughts like a herd of elephants;

there were plenty of opportunities. What was the use anyway, she reasoned, contracting a really good case of self-pity.

Noticing apathetic feelings and realizing Jean was probably on the verge of breaking her diet, her friends began suggesting remedies outside of food as a rescue from certain doom.

"Get your hair done," one said.

"Let's go shopping," another suggested.

"A good movie will take your mind off your problems."

"Talk to the doctors in the morning. They will know what to do."

In no mood to have her hair done, to see a movie, or to go shopping, wanting only to be left alone, Jean recognized an old familiar habit, isolation. One of the suggestions had, however, made an impression; she saw the medical director the next morning. Her chart showed good structure, normal blood pressure, and her walking regime of ten to twelve miles a day. The doctor asked numerous questions about her general health and feelings, and suggested a decrease in her calorie intake if she felt able to handle it. Jean was willing to try anything at this point, and they worked out a plan of what to cut to get the maximum protein: three egg whites instead of six for breakfast, a bowl of soup for lunch without the salad or meat, and one-half portion of meat for dinner with one vegetable, a beverage with each meal. Her daily walking regime was to remain the same. If this change in food intake made her too tired to walk, her new diet would have to be reevaluated.

The therapist agreed with this idea and made a few additional suggestions: she was to buy a tape measure—usually when the scale doesn't budge, inches are coming off; go out and do something special—buy bubblebath; get her hair set; look at herself in the mirror more often; shop for new outfits and try on clothes. The weight loss would become evident as she graduated to smaller sizes. He cautioned her to dress immediately upon rising in the morning instead of lolling around in pajamas, and to keep the clothes on until bedtime, so she would be ready for any social opportunity that might come along. Agreeing to think more about personal appearance and less of the scale, Jean headed to the store for a tape measure. She started the new regime the next meal.

Her body didn't take long to adjust to the lower calorie intake, and after a few days the weight began to drop steadily. She discussed this later with the doctor, who suggested that perhaps her body did not require much food. At times she discovered she lost weight more slowly and instead lost inches. The therapist's suggestion of looking in mirrors more often was excellent. Jean had still been thinking of herself as the obese person she was at the beginning of the program, but the lady in the mirror made her aware of the weight loss. Vanity behavior began to develop also: she took more time to apply makeup in the mornings, experimenting with eye shadow and different hair styles to complement her changing facial contours. All of this readjustment gave her a greater awareness of herself as an individual, and her accomplishments supplied a greater determination to continue building a better Jean.

* * *

FRIENDSHIP! How beautiful and important this word is, not only for our everyday living, but to help us over the humps dietwise. As you have read, without friends, Jean's despair may have carried her down the road to ruin. Instead, her friends became her sounding board, her mental boost, her companion, and, momentarily, her strength. A give-and-take relationship between two people can be most rewarding emotionally and structurally. As two of the best long-standing friends, we can recommend this fellowship most heartily and enthusiastically.

Another thing we need to stress is that no two people are alike. What is good for you may not be so for someone else. Unfortunately, Jean discovered her body's requirement for food was very small. Therefore, it was most important that she seek medical advice, not only on cutting calories, but in establishing a balanced diet to encompass her daily requirements of vitamins, minerals, and iron. Once she understood and accepted her unfortunate circumstance, she was able to cope with her problem. You too may need fewer calories to lose weight. If you *have* remained structured, and your weight loss during the past eight or nine days has been nil, talk with your doctor. He will help you find the cause and will guide you from there. Remember, you are striving for a *healthier* as well as happier you.

CHAPTER XI

Self-reverence, self-knowledge,
self-control,
These three alone lead life to
sovereign power.
ALFRED, LORD TENNYSON

Em spent many days recounting the details of her mother's visit to all her friends on the diet program. The stories were repeated numerous times to everyone, and the joy of success was shared by all.

"I was very assertive," Em told them, "especially when I asked Mum not to buy me any clothes now. It surprised me that assertiveness could also be for the other person. I had never thought of assertiveness as being applied to anything except for getting something *you* want. This time it was the other way around, and it was just as difficult to do. I realize now I had always felt guilty about asking my parents *not* to do something for me, as well as asking them *for* a favor."

"Some people don't know what's good for them. If

someone's sick, but refuses to acknowledge it, you must be assertive to make him stay in bed."

"I never thought of it that way," another remarked. "Assertiveness can be applied to something that will be good for the other person, too."

"That's why I told Toni I wouldn't drive her to the dining room in the mornings. We both need to walk, and when she starts walking, she'll lose better, and in turn feel better, as I do. Now we both will get that added exercise," Jean said.

"When I want to walk, I ask people in the dining room to walk with me," Lee recounted, "but if they sit and talk for hours, and I want to go, I get up and leave. Is that being aggressive?"

"No, you're not hurting them by leaving, you're only helping yourself. By staying with them, you might have been persuaded not to walk at all, which would have hurt you. But you could ask them again before leaving, and tell them when you want to walk. Either way, by leaving or by urging the others to walk with you, you are being assertive," one old timer answered, and everyone agreed.

"I wrote my parents an assertive letter a while back," Em told them. "We had planned to go to Hawaii for spring vacation this year. When I decided to come here they wanted to cancel their plans. My parents needed a rest from the grind, so I wrote, urging them to go on without me, saying I wouldn't take no for an answer."

"Did they go?"

"No, being stubborn, they refused to go without me. I tried, though, and they appreciated it. My father has planned to give my mother an anniversary present of a cruise through the Greek Islands because he now knows that I don't mind their going without me."

"Trying to help others is a form of assertiveness, if it benefits you or not, I gather then," another newcomer remarked.

Jean replied, "Yes, sometimes if you want to do something for yourself, it can be very beneficial to others, too. I write most of the checks at home, and when my husband or daughter wants to buy something we can't afford, I explain my reason for denying them the money. My husband agreed to let me handle the money in the first place because he knows I have a good sense for wise spending.

"It doesn't have to be an individual thing, though. It doesn't have to deny one person one thing to benefit the other. At parties, for instance, if you cook the meal you will serve salt-free or salt-poor, you benefit by being able to eat with everyone else, and you benefit the guests because salt isn't good for anyone. They can always add their own at the table if they wish. You aren't denying yourself or them the right to have a good time."

"Speaking of parties," one friend piped in, "is anyone going to the party at the Hilton tonight? Susan and her husband are giving a farewell party . . . they are leaving the program on Sunday."

"I wonder what they'll serve," mused one.

"We'll see when we get there, I guess. I hope it's nothing delicious. I don't want to have to ward off temptation all evening. That makes it no fun for me," another declared.

The evening came and many dieters went to the Hilton, not knowing what to expect. In the middle of the room was a table decorated with a large wine cooler, necks of wine bottles sticking out. Around the silver wine coolers were trays of beautifully decorated hors d'oeuvres: cucumber slices, carrot sticks, celery sticks, radishes, grapefruit and orange sections. Everything was structured, and there, lounging comfortably in the corner, talking to a dieter, glass of low-sodium wine in hand, sat the program director. Next to him, looking equally regal, lounged the therapist. The medical director was out of town, they learned later.

The evening was very enjoyable. Everyone nibbled on the hors d'oeuvres, talked avidly about everything—from diet to weight, of course. Pictures were taken of smiling dieters; many had been "dry" for quite a while and one glass of wine proved plenty. Soft music played in the background, everyone was comfortable with one another, and the party broke up quite late. Susan had been very assertive, serving only foods acceptable on their diet, thereby helping everyone and making the atmosphere relaxed and enjoyable. Assertiveness, they were learning, *is* beneficial to all.

* * *

In practicing assertiveness, the key is to think of yourself in relation to others. An assertive decision should not be totally self-centered. Certainly you must consider your needs and act accordingly, feel positive about any decision made, and be confident once a conclusion has been reached. As you may already have learned, there is a thin line between non-assertiveness, assertiveness, and aggressiveness. Learning the distinction requires much thought, planning, and practice *before* the application, as Em discovered when anticipating her mother's visit. You must become adept at not letting people walk all over you and, on the other hand, guard against walking over people with whom *you* come in contact. No doubt you are saying, "This is easier said than done," and you're so right. Regrettably, this cannot be learned overnight. But remember, like all habits, practice makes perfect—and we are still practicing! We have found, however, that most of our decisions can be made more easily and more swifly. And we are happier because of this ability. PRACTICE, it *will* come!

CHAPTER XII

Beauty stands
In the admiration only of weak minds
Led captive.
JOHN MILTON

One day Em was peering into store windows, checking out the latest styles, styles that she, after losing twenty pounds, would be wearing. It was a nice day, the sun was shining, and everything seemed right with the world. Em smiled, seeing a dress that very much appealed to her.

"Excuse me, could you tell me where Fayetteville Street is?"

Spinning around, startled by the voice so close behind her, Em saw a man smiling at her, a quizzical look on his face. Relaxing, one hand on her hip and the other pointing toward downtown, Em smiled at the man, "I'm not sure, but I think it's down that way, running parallel to this street, about eight or nine blocks from here."

"You have nice breasts, lady!"

71

Horrified, completely at a loss for words, she spun around and walked fast without direction. She fought brimming tears. Why would he say that to me? Had she led him on? She hated him, wanted to cry, wanted someone with whom to talk. Finally she started talking to herself for lack of companionship and, after drawing a few deep breaths, averted her thoughts. Now, what did that dress cost? What did it look like? Oh yes, she remembered. Lost in her thoughts of the dress, she found peace of mind.

Later Em found Ann in the dining room and talked to her about the incident. "I just can't seem to come up with the right response fast enough. I thought of the right reaction about three hours after it happened. I wish I could think faster; I got myself really worked up over it because I didn't have the right comeback. Had I been able to think of the suitable response on the spot, I never would have given it another thought."

"Don't worry about it, Em," Ann consoled her. "That's one of our faults as non-assertive people: we can never think of the right words until much too late. We haven't defended ourselves in so long that we have forgotten how, or we might never have learned. Only practice will solve that, which is why we are here. It's situations like that which have caused many of us to become obese, so in order to conquer our obesity, we must solve the problems at their roots, like killing weeds. It's just a matter of time and practice.

"I'll tell you what the therapist told me to do," she said. "First, get the facts clear in your mind. What exactly did he say to you? Write it down. Write down what you said and did after his remark, and then write down what you should have said and done. Next, start practicing, first in front of a mirror. When you can see that you are saying what you ought to have said with the right body position, expression, voice control, and attitude, write out a script with these things on it. Practice gestures, timing, and, most important, eye contact. Once you have mastered this alone, ask a trusted friend to rehearse the script with you. Ask her opinion of what you said and the way you said it. She'll give you some helpful hints on how to improve your response. You have to do this often since practice is the most important thing for us, and you'll be able to think of responses in these situations faster. It does take time, though. You can't expect to be able to make a good comeback remark in the next situation that requires one."

"But what if you know the person and they said something that didn't sit right with you, but you couldn't think of how to put your own feelings into words?"

"If the situation was important to you, you should call them when you've practiced the correct response and feel certain of yourself. Next, face them and tell them how you feel in person."

"If that works, I sure am going to thank you, Ann!"

"Don't thank me, Em, thank the person you are assertive with. If it works, they won't do it again."

"I really appreciate your help. I had just about decided it wasn't worth the effort to diet and get that kind of remark. I don't want to wear anything fitted around here anymore."

"But you should Em. With your new figure, you should start pampering yourself and look your best. Buy some new makeup and, for goodness sake, get a new pair of pants! The ones you're wearing must be about four sizes too big and look terrible. Now that you're getting close to goal, you'll find getting dressed up makes you feel better, and it makes you and others see how pretty you are. All that fat hid your beauty for too many years."

Laughing and teasing, they walked out to Pineapplehead to bid him good evening.

* * *

Em has just brought out what most obese people have forgotten, or perhaps have never learned—how to handle a compliment. Her experience was, to say the least, horrifying, and fortunately she was taught ways of overcoming situations such as this.

This experience, however, does provide us with an opportunity to zero in on how to cope with an honest-to-goodness genuine physical compliment. Reactions can be anything from stammering to blushing to running. Jean's first reaction when brought face to face with a hearty congratulations complete with approving eye appraisal from the opposite sex was fear. Why? Simply, that for the many years she had carried around those one hundred extra pounds, an experience of this kind passed her by. Suddenly, like Em, she was brought

73

face to face with a situation she could not handle. Thus, fear! Em was thrust into an incident that demanded more than just "directions," and she too experienced momentary fear.

And the antonym of fear? . . . confidence, courage, calmness. In other words, *practice* over and over if necessary as Em was instructed. Each day throughout your dieting, new events will show themselves. Begin now, learning how to handle each one as it comes. And each new happening conquered will bring with it confidence and strength to face and overcome the next.

CHAPTER XIII

The ear of jealousy heareth all things.
WISDOM OF SOLOMON

At ten pounds from her goal weight, Em's excitement increased. Her mother and sister would be coming in two weeks to spend a few days and then all three would fly back to their home in Connecticut for a week. She was beginning to look normal, and the compliments increased every day. Em was happy and showed it.

Walking downtown one day a passing car tooted at her followed by a loud wolf whistle. Her first reaction was the same as it had always been, revulsion. People always make fun of fat people. Then realizing she wasn't fat any more, she wondered why she was still getting the sarcastic whistles. Bringing this up in group, she was assured by her friends that the whistle was complimentary. It would take some time before the immediate reaction of disgust and embarrassment would go away, and Em would have to change her reaction as the intention behind the action itself changed. She was upset nonetheless, and felt an undercurrent all week in the dining room which had been bothering her. The feeling was in the room at that moment and she realized that others were looking at her with mild jealousy.

Once she recognized it, she noticed it more and more and, thinking back, could remember other comments in the dining room that had shown a hint of jealousy also. The tension mounted in the room until Em could bear it no longer.

"I have a question," she burst out. "Why is it that I get the distinct feeling of hostility lately? I feel as if people are jealous because I am near goal or something. How can I overcome this feeling? It's driving me crazy. I feel as if I won't be able to stand another minute in the dining room at times. How can I make people realize that I am still going through the same things they are? I haven't been unstructured, and I have been exercising faithfully and good loss has been my reward. What right have others to be jealous of me if they haven't tried as hard as I have or haven't been on the program as long or have more to lose? There isn't any basis for comparison. And yet they seem to be comparing."

"That's because you've changed your attitude!" another yelled back. "I don't think it's nice for anyone to talk about anyone else behind their back."

"What do you mean? What have I said about you?"

"I've heard a rumor that you were talking at a table about other people on the program, myself included, and saying whether or not you thought they had lost weight."

Em was shocked, but knew instantly to what she was referring. She remembered a friend telling her of the table conversation: one person had been talking about everyone else on the program saying that so and so went off the diet yesterday, and so and so gained four pounds this morning, and another person didn't seem to have lost anything in two weeks, saying the information came from Em.

Em forced herself back to the present and the hurled accusations. She had never before been able to take criticism, tuning out to what was being said, thereby not benefiting from suggestions. This time, however, she forced herself to listen. The criticism was misplaced, she knew, but couldn't bring herself to say so. Instead she simply told the girl she was sorry, offering no other comment. Em realized later she still had a great deal to learn. She had been used as a doormat again and hadn't defended herself. She made amends by apologizing. She had lost a battle that she hadn't even been involved in. The therapist's words, however, did keep ringing in her ears: she must concentrate on her successes and not her failures. Yes, she had made a step in the right direction by learning to listen objectively to criticism. With more practice she would be able to handle such situations fully. Practice was what was needed most. And practice she did.

Jean had a similar experience. Upon entering the program she naturally became close to her rooming-house friend, Betty. They shared cars, experiences, clothes, and became constant companions. A former dieter, Pat, returning to the program, telephoned Betty asking her to meet her at the airport. Jean and Betty had made previous plans and did not want to disrupt their structured day. Betty told Pat she would not be able to come, but that there was a limousine service from the airport into town.

Calling when she arrived, Pat asked if Betty knew of any available rooms for rent. That day she moved into a lovely home two blocks away from their house, and Pat assumed she would be included in their outings since she had no car.

Not wanting to be tied down, Betty did not encourage this arrangement and she and Jean continued their structured daily life. Pat was included and invited whenever time schedules coincided and the three walked frequently to Pineapplehead sharing their experiences.

It wasn't long before Jean sensed Pat's jealousy of her friendship with Betty. At this same time she was beginning to get feedback from friends in the dining room about untrue rumors. Jean's immediate reaction was to withdraw, to not appear in the dining room. Several close friends became aware of her feelings and arranged a pre-breakfast walk. She joined them and was helped tremendously, knowing this was her friends' way of saying they were behind her and knew there was no truth to any of the rumors. They stayed together all day, walking, sharing experiences, and eating. Their love gave her the strength, encouragement, and determination to put things in their proper perspective. Their assertiveness enabled Jean to realize that other close associates who knew her well realized the rumors were just idle gossip and did not let them influence their friendship.

By her friends' assertiveness Jean overcame Pat's jealousy and her own feelings of withdrawal, but realized that in future situations she must assert herself and face her own problems. She might not have close friends around to draw strength from. She too had a great deal of practicing to do in order to learn how to live the assertive way.

* * *

Let us reflect for a moment on the word *normal*. There is a great distinction between looking normal, and normal eating. Now is a good time to again emphasize: An obese person is always obese. Alcohol is and always will be a No-No for a non-practicing alcoholic just as fatty, greasy foods are and always will be a No-No for the obese. Begin right now to stop kidding yourself. When goal is reached you will *not* be able to eat anything and everything. You have been learning and practicing correct eating techniques which include preparing a nutritionally balanced diet that your doctor recommended. When you reach goal your daily intake can be somewhat augmented and some foods can be supplemented, but your balanced diet will remain your *foundation* for sound eating. Perhaps this expression will put our point in perspective for you: WE EAT TO LIVE, NOT LIVE TO EAT!

Another point that needs mentioning is that now you are losing weight and substituting more constructive habits for bad ones, and this is a good opportunity to stop for a few minutes and observe the changing you. You are undergoing an inward as well as outward transformation, aren't you? You are becoming more aware of things around you, more confident of yourself, able to analyze things more clearly, and are observing things in a more colorful light. Like us, you are experiencing some of the greatest rewards for successful dieting, and we rejoice with you. Perhaps you have found there are times when it is difficult to let go of old habits, old ways of doing things. Perhaps you are experiencing, as Em did, others' envy of your success so far. Occurrences of this type, unfortunately, can happen and you must prepare yourself to overcome them. How? Concentrate on your objectives: health, happiness, beauty. Let nothing stand in the way of building a better you!

CHAPTER XIV

To be prepared for war is one of the
most effectual means of
preserving peace.
GEORGE WASHINGTON

Having been on the program for four months, Jean planned to return home for the week of her daughter's graduation from college. And, nearing her goal weight, Em planned a short visit home also. Both began preparations by moving into the homebound behavioral therapy group, which adapts behavior learned on the program to the home environment. They discussed some of the points mentioned during their afternoon walk.

"Em, I think it's a good idea to browse through the supermarkets a few times before we start shopping, to get used to the prices and the food environment again. After four months, I have no idea what a loaf of bread costs."

"You buy a loaf of bread and the doctors will have your

head! Remember what they told us: 'Bread is the shaft of life.'" Laughing, she continued, "I do need to frequent the stores to practice passing by the goodies. It'll be automatic for me to head for all the bad stuff."

"We'll have to make sure we don't carry any money for the first few visits."

"Jean, I'm not even sure which stores at home carry diet foods. It could be that none do, since we don't live near any big cities."

"Let's go to all the stores here and make a note of which ones carry diet food. If you buy some things here, they'll see you through until you can find a store at home that carries them."

"Maybe I'd better write home and send a list of the brand names and foods I'll need, and have my parents check the stores for me. Then, when Mum and my sister come down here for the two days before we all fly home, they can tell me what the stores don't carry, and we can stock up here."

"I'm going to have a problem adjusting to supermarkets. I'll be buying food for the whole family, not just for me," Jean commented.

"I don't have to go into any stores at home if I don't want to; Mum will buy my food for me when she does her normal shopping. But, when I return I plan to stay on the program for two weeks and then cook for myself in my apartment for a month. I'm going to have to learn how to shop. This will be a valuable experience as I'll be cooking for myself all through college from now on."

"Maybe I'll make a contract with my family: I'll ask them to buy their own goodies, which will make the shopping easier."

"What will you give them in return, Jean?"

"I don't know yet. Whatever they want . . . we'll have to work that out when I get home."

"You have it easier than me though, Jean, because you'll be buying meat and staples in reasonably normal quantities. I'll have to buy the smallest packages I can find, and probably still will have waste and leftovers."

"My problem is going to be those leftovers, Em. Tom was raised on a farm and I've learned from his mother to cook huge portions for lunch and serve the leftovers for supper. I can't do that any more; I'll eat them all afternoon just like I used to. I'll have to learn to cook proportionately, and only one meal at a time."

"I'll have to cook for one person. I enjoy cooking gourmet style, with herbs and spices, but I derive most pleasure from other people's enjoyment of my cooking. Cooking for myself alone doesn't enthuse me much."

"I've never learned to cook with herbs and spices. My seasoning consists of ham hocks, bacon, salt, and pepper. How about writing some of your recipes down for me?"

"Jean, why don't you come off the program with me when you come back? We can plan our menus together and I won't have to cook for just one person."

"That sounds fabulous, Em, but you'd be getting the raw end of the deal. You do all the cooking, and I reap all the recipes. How about me being chief bottle washer?"

"You're not getting out of cooking that easily, Jean. You and I will be eating entirely different things for breakfast and lunch, since you'll still be on your present diet, and I'll be eating more, so you can cook your own egg whites and soup yourself. We'll race to see who gets to wash up. At dinner, though, I'll cook a meal we both can have, and you are more than welcome to clean up the mess."

"Thanks loads! Hope you don't mess up the whole kitchen. Em, with the different calorie counts, we'll have to buy proportionately. Otherwise our grocery bill will be sky high. What we could do is plan menus for the whole week, estimate the cost and halve the bill. Not paying any on the electric bill should balance out your increase of food."

"That will save us both money."

"We're going to have to make the grocery list out on a full stomach. If I made the list now, I'd buy the store out. My hunger alarm clock is ringing." Jean looked at her watch. "Eleven-thirty. We'd better double time it back to the dining room."

They walked on in silence, both weighing the pros and cons of the proposed arrangements. "Let's think about this, Em. I'll have to check with the doctors and get their approval. We do have three more weeks."

* * *

The important words in this chapter are *preparation* and *planning*. How many times have you gone to the refrigerator around 6:00 P.M., opened the door, and thought, "Let's see, what can I fix for supper tonight?" Dangerous, isn't it?

A friend phones and announces, "That movie we have been waiting for is playing at the Center . . . I'll pick you up in half an hour," and after investigating, you find that what you want to wear needs washing! No time to eat—you'll just grab something.

Or perhaps you walk in the room and overhear your spouse inviting those unexpected guests to join you for the evening meal.

Of course, you can add many such circumstances to these, and you will find that in most situations a little planning, a little preparation beforehand, would have seen you through. Plan your menus ahead, have the outfit ready just in case, put aside that extra dollar or two, have an extra portion or two of fish or steak in the freezer. Believe us, a few moments of planning and preparation today will save you much frustration tomorrow.

CHAPTER XV

Be not the first by whom
the new are tried,
Nor yet the last to lay the old aside.
ALEXANDER POPE

Realizing that she would be going home soon, Em made her meal plans and grocery list and sent them to her mother who wrote back saying she would be glad to do the shopping for her first two days so that the right foods would be in the house when she arrived. "Now what problems will I encounter at home?" Em began thinking of her old habits. She had a tendency to eat after the meal was over by cleaning off the plates, putting the scraps in her disposal mouth, and then taking hunks of leftover roast and vegetables as a final course. If there were only a few mouthfuls of vegetables left, or only a roll or two, she would also dispose of them the neatest way—who noticed a few more pounds? Realizing this behavior would have to change, she again wrote her parents stating she would gladly do the dishes if someone else would clean the plates and put the leftovers away before she started washing. An agreement was made.

The trip home was important to Em; it was her first since she had started the program and she wanted her arrival to be a family secret. New clothes were needed badly. She had no idea what size she was now since she still wore her size eighteens. She decided to wait before buying anything until her mother could be with her to shop. Meanwhile she began looking around. One day she decided to try on a dress. To her great joy she found herself in a size ten! Unable to resist, she bought the dress and two others, all three on sale.

The day Em's mother and sister arrived, Em was four pounds from her goal. Thirty-five pounds had been lost since her mother's last visit, and her sister hadn't seen her since she left home. The excitement was almost unbearable. She decided to buy a pantsuit that she had had her eye on for a week, and wear it to the airport. She was tempted to wear it inside out so the size tag would show, but Jean squelched that idea.

That evening Jean drove Em to the airport and dropped her off; her mother and sister would rent a car for their stay. She spied them at the car rental counter. Taking a deep breath, Em strolled over to her family and said, "Excuse me." A few shocked seconds later there were oohs and aahs and tears all around, everyone talking at once. Laughing, they got the keys to the car and headed into town. The rest of the evening was spent making plans for the next day's shopping venture. Em showed her mother the three dresses she had bought and told her of her decision to buy everything else when she came. There was a great deal to be done before they all went home in two days. It was agreed they would say nothing to Em's father on the phone about Em's success. She had not told her family anything about her weight, and they had therefore no idea she was close to goal. What a surprise she had in store for those back home!

The next morning three giggling ladies climbed into the car and headed for the shopping mall. For Em, a new wardrobe! Almost everything tried on was bought since everything looked well on her. Shopping was a whole new experience now for Em, and the three acted like children buying their first clothes. Em wanted to buy a bathing suit for the summer and had already seen a one-piece suit she liked. Her sister urged her to try a two-piece.

"Me?" Em exclaimed in mock horror. "I couldn't possibly wear a two-piece. There isn't enough material to cover all of me. I'd hang out all over the place. Imagine!"

"I am, Sis, here, try this on."

Em couldn't believe her eyes. It fit, and what's more looked beautiful on her—no bulges anywhere. One more purchase was thus added to the growing stack. Despite chiding from her mother, Em found herself looking at dark colors and slimming lines from habit. It was hard to realize she no longer needed these camouflages.

Lunch was eaten at 11:30, right on schedule for Em as planned. They ate at the cafeteria in the mall and Em ordered a salad; her mother and sister, broiled fish with all the trimmings. "The next time we eat here," Em joyfully exclaimed, "I will eat the broiled mackerel and *you* will eat the salad." Lunch was a very happy occasion and discussion prevailed about the loot they had bagged and would bag after lunch.

A bit tired, but no less determined, they set out once again buying shorts, slacks, skirts, dresses, and blouses. Em's mother handed her a halter to try on. Em looked at it and then her mother in horror.

"I'd feel naked!" she exclaimed, wondering where her mother's conservative tastes had gone.

"Oh, come on, try it. I used to wear the three-cornered scarves myself," her mother told her laughing at Em's expression.

The halter was purchased along with other short blouses exposing much more than Em was used to. At the end of the day Em realized she had bought no shirts that covered her middle. "If you don't have a spare tire any more," they teased, "flaunt it!"

The evening was spent at the steakhouse outside of town where Em and her mother had eaten on her previous visit. The evening was very enjoyable and the meal went well. No comments were made about either weight or diet and Em was relieved.

The next day was spent shopping for things they had forgotten—shoes, purse, and necessities for home. The day was much more leisurely spent and everything on the list was bought. Dinner that night was shared with two of Em's close friends.

Returning to the apartment all three began packing for their trip home. To surprise her father, the happy three decided to fly home four hours earlier than planned, arriving just before a Board of Governor's meeting of the local country club, which was to be held at their house.

They were able to change their flight reservations, and arrived just before noon. They all gobbled a quick lunch, anxious to arrive home before the meeting started, and made it with five minutes to spare. Parking on the main road, Em got out and walked across the lawn to where her father was talking to an early arrival.

"Excuse me, could you tell me where the Recorder Center is?" she asked her father, owner of the business located next door to their home.

"You've come to the right place," he said, face stern, looking her straight in the eye.

"Oh. Well . . . I, I'm . . . ah, looking for a recorder." Em had not anticipated her father's not recognizing her. He started to ask her to come into the office, then did a double take. Em burst into a huge grin.

"My God, what are you doing home?" and gave her the biggest of bear hugs. Em knew the man standing with her father, but he hadn't the slightest notion of whom she was. The situation was utterly perfect.

Em's mother and sister had peered through the trees to watch the happy reunion. The four of them decided to have some fun and introduce Em to the governors, all of whom were close family friends, as her mother's cousin Mary who had just flown in. One of Em's closest friends, Pat, would be there and she wondered how far the deception would go.

On entering the house Em experienced a strong revival of an old habit. The atmosphere triggered an instant thought— a whiskey sour. Before, her first job upon arriving home from any trip had been to mix drinks. This behavior must come to an end, she realized. She dismissed the fatal idea and went in to meet the board members.

"Cousin Mary" was introduced to their neighbor from across the street and then to Pat. "How do you do," Pat said.

86

Speaking to Em's father she said, "You know, she looks very much like . . . I don't believe it!" Tears and peals of laughter from all who had gathered around followed. All were deeply impressed by Em's success and everyone complimented her with oohs and aahs.

That evening Em was found in the kitchen cooking her own meal. An agreement had been made with her parents that she would eat at her regularly scheduled times since her short visit did not permit her time to adjust to later meal hours to which her family was accustomed. She ate in the kitchen and followed her red and white commandments strictly. Her parents expressed their wish that she at least sit with them while they ate their dinner at 7:30. Em also agreed to do all the dishes after they had finished dinner. Her mother had already worked out a system for the removal of scraps and leftovers as Em had asked in her letter. From the first meal, everything worked well and life remained structured.

The first morning home the scale showed Em that she had reached goal. She ran downstairs and spread the news.

"Does this mean you're off the diet?" her family asked.

"No, I plan to stay on my regular eating routine until I return to the program. I will cut down on my walking while I'm home, though, and let my body get used to less exercise."

"It's a good thing," her father laughingly commented as he glanced out the window. In her excitement, she had neglected to look outside. It was snowing—in May! She discovered it was twenty-seven degrees outside and she had to walk in it. Cringing, she ate her breakfast *very* slowly.

Despite the snow, Em bundled up in her father's winter jacket and trudged around a two-mile stretch her parents had clocked for her. She did this after each meal, totaling a meager six miles each day, a bare pittance compared to the sixteen she had been doing. She planned to decrease her walking even more when she started maintenance to make her exercise more consistent with what she would be doing at college.

Em made certain she always had something to do that interested her enough to require all of her attention, as she remembered her weakest moments had always been the idle ones. When she wasn't walking and cooking she unpacked the suitcase full of unwanted and unnecessary things she had brought home. Most went to the Salvation Army; some went to a New York clothing exchange. She went through all her old clothes and threw away everything that didn't fit perfectly . . . which turned out to be everything she owned, except for her new wardrobe.

Her sister had to lend her a dress to wear that night to the dinner party they all had been invited to that evening. Em decided to eat at home, however, and participate only in conversation and coffee that evening. She called her hostess and explained her situation, and Mrs. Westover welcomed her to join them nevertheless. Dinner at the Westover's was a very welcome experience for Em. The other guests didn't know her well, therefore did not realize she had been dieting, and no mention was made of it.

The meal was served Oriental style, complete with chopsticks. In the middle of the table was a huge pot with a chimney protruding from the center. The chimney base was filled with hot coals from the fireplace and the pot was filled with boiling chicken broth. Each person was passed plates of raw vegetables, raw meat, and fish which they held in the broth for a few seconds until cooked. Em had not been looking forward to sitting at the table watching everyone else eat. So she passed everyone the raw meats and vegetables, making sure that not one plate was empty. She refilled side dishes of rice and serving platters when they were low. This provided much enjoyment for her, as well as exercise, and was greatly appreciated by her hostess. Without Em she would have had to do all the passing herself. The meal was finished and Em realized she had not once had time to sit down at the table.

While the other guests were eating dessert, Em cleared the table and rinsed the dishes. She did have coffee with the others after dinner and, for that short time, relaxed. The minute she sat down, however, she discovered she was extremely tired and looked forward to going home. Her parents, not being on Em's meager diet, of course could not understand her exhaustion and had no thoughts of leaving. Em finally managed to pull them away and, once home, gratefully crawled into bed.

At dinner the next evening Em decided to discuss her summer plans, after she finished maintenance, with her family.

"Mum and Dad, I'd like to go to Boston for the summer," she started. "I'd like to take a secretarial course there and live in an apartment. What are your thoughts?"

"That sounds like a good idea," her father said, which gave her the courage to go further.

"I won't be making any money, so I'll have to rely on you to support me. I'd take a job, but I won't be there for more than two months and I doubt I'd even find a job in that length of time."

"You will need a typing course, and it will stand you in good stead always. We'd be willing to support you if you'd like to do it."

She decided to assert herself a bit more since the response had been surprisingly positive. "I'll need the car to take my stuff up, and I'll bring it home the first weekend."

"That sounds like the best solution," they agreed. It had been so easy! Never before would Em have dared be so frank. She thought of all the miserable days and months she had spent, wanting something but never asking for it. This opened a whole new way of life to her, and an entirely new relationship with her parents: loving and solid.

The next evening Em was invited to Joan and Tilly's for after dinner coffee. She observed their eating habits to see if the reason for Tilly's lack of a weight problem was the same as her mother's. Amazed, she saw Tilly follow the red and white commandments to the letter, even though she had never seen them. When Tilly had finished, leaving a bite of everything on her plate, Em exclaimed, "Now I know the secret!"

"To what?" Tilly asked surprised.

"You waited before you started eating, you took at least twenty minutes to eat, you laid down your fork between every bite, and you left some on your plate. No wonder you're so skinny."

"I never even noticed how I ate before. I was taught to eat this way, I guess."

"Yes, she was," Tilly's mother answered. "I have tried to teach my children to eat slowly. None of them have ever had a weight problem."

The days had warmed up considerably and Em continued her two-mile walk after each meal. She had planned all her meals in advance and structured all her activities so carefully that she found she had just enough time to do everything and was never bored. Not once during her stay did she find time for television, her greatest downfall in the past. She remembered getting a beer at most commercial breaks and finishing off a large bag of potato chips per night. If she watched television during the day, she devoured peanut butter sandwiches as well. She decided the best thing to do would be to structure television completely out of her day, and it worked.

Contracts had been made, problems overcome, old friends introduced to the new Em, and everything went well. The family was pleased and friends overjoyed. "Just don't gain it back" seemed to be one of the prominent remarks which irritated Em to some extent, but she found she could handle this. If she could make it this far, she certainly would never go back to her old life. The few days at home had reinforced her determination never to gain any weight back. Life was beautiful and there to be enjoyed, something Em had experienced rarely before. She wouldn't let anyone else down because she wasn't going to let herself down. She had become increasingly aware, back in the old environment, that the main thing to be changed was her own attitude. For years she had lived for everyone but herself. Now she must live for herself first, and she had taken a big step in that direction. She was pleased and proud, and looked forward to going back to the program to learn more, so that her life henceforth would be the most fruitful possible.

On her last day at home, Em took all the lists she had prepared for things she would return with, and consulted her mother. "Take anything you need from my herb cabinet, Em. I can always get more," her mother offered. Em helped herself and loaded her suitcase with jars of various shapes and sizes. In the attic she found her set of dishes she had bought that fall at college but never used. The prospect of putting them to good use was appealing, especially when the things that would one day go on them were considered. Her mother gave her a set of silverware to use and surprised her with a set of ovenproof casseroles. Em asked her mother about the possibilities of an electric blender and a slow cooker, and her wishes were immediately granted. "I don't know why I didn't think of that before," her mother told her. "Of course you'll need the blender. The slow cooker will be great fun for you to experiment with, and I'll gladly give it to you if you promise to try lots of new recipes and write them all down for me. I'll order the appliances right away and have them sent to you."

Another contract made, mother and daughter both showed their happiness. The excitement of Em's first kitchen and her new life ahead had brought the two much closer and they discovered a deep love for one another which had rarely surfaced before. Grinning from ear to ear and laughing over her mother's stories of her first kitchen, Em and her mother packed and planned furiously. Cookbooks, both diet and gourmet, were "stolen" from her mother's kitchen and packed. "I want those recipes you invent, remember," her mother reminded her. "That's my part of the contract, if you want all these cookbooks." Em assured her she would return with many new recipes and also threatened, "Better watch it, Mum, or I'll become a better cook than you!"

Em left that afternoon, saying goodbye to parents far dearer to her than she had ever known before. Settling back in the plane she thought about the changes in the environment at home and it suddenly dawned on her: the atmosphere hadn't changed a bit; she had, drastically. Her new life had already started, and she didn't even have to leave her hometown to begin.

* * *

The first thing you have noted from this chapter, we hope, is Em's planning. Whether the situations she experienced are similar to your own or not is unimportant. Whatever your circumstance, preparation is necessary for attaining and maintaining your goal. If you will notice, all through these many events Em remained one step ahead, and thus was able to remain calm, cool, and collected. See how it works?

May we also stress Em's answer to her family's question, "Does this mean you're off the diet?" Their question so naturally implied: Hurrah, you've done it, you're now a normal human being, your problems are over. STOP! Believe us, if you agreed with this and ate accordingly, within a week's time your scale would register close to ten pounds heavier! When goal is reached, you are simply ready for the next phase: maintenance. And without this important step, the weight *will* climb again. No, you're not through. As we emphasized in the Introduction, the tendency towards obesity for a person with a weight problem is *always* present; it can, however, be controlled. Let us teach you how!

CHAPTER XVI

Attempt the end, and never stand to
doubt; Nothing's so hard, but search
will find it out.
ROBERT HERRICK

Jean met Em at the airport. The extra cartons Em had
brought with her aroused Jean's curiosity. "You'll see when
we get home," Em mysteriously chided. Reaching Em's apartment, they unpacked the cumbersome cartons and Em
proudly showed Jean her new dishes, cookware, and piles of
cookbooks, arousing great excitement in them both over the
rapidly approaching experience off service.

Em was now ready to start maintenance and had been
thinking on the plane about her food allowance increase.

"Em, just what is maintenance? You've reached your goal.
Can't you just watch what you eat and the scale from now
on?"

"The way the doctors described it to me, I've got to slowly
build my calorie intake up to a level that will satisfy my

suppressed cravings and at the same time reach that point where I will neither gain nor lose. The process must be slow so my body can readjust, and they cautioned me that it may take weeks before I find my own level. It may be 1200, 1500, or even 2000 calories a day. Once I see how much I can eat, I should be able to judge without counting calories. Just weighing once a week should tell me whether I'm maintaining my balance. And too, Jean, I want to adjust my present diet to one that I can live with for the rest of my life.

"Tight seams would also give you a checking point for maintenance," added Jean thoughtfully.

"Wow, my parents would have my head! But not only that, Jean, I feel like a new person now. I've been given a new lease on life. I don't ever want to go back to rock bottom."

"We won't, Em. We both must keep looking up! How are you to start maintenance? I'll be starting soon myself, so tell all."

"The doctors have suggested I begin by adding 200 calories daily." Eagerly she told Jean of her plans for the extras. "I think what I'll do is increase breakfast and lunch, leaving my dinner allotment alone because that satisfies me now."

The next day Em started her new regimen and was ecstatic. All that food! It was unbelievable. Her stomach hadn't shrunk as she thought, and she ate every mouthful with great gusto. The second morning, however, brought her close to tears: she had gained a pound and a half. She ran for help; her first thoughts were of food, a signal of doom! Smiling at her fears, the doctors told her a momentary weight gain was to be expected when increasing her intake. Soon her body would readjust to the increased calories and she would then start losing again. When this happened she would be able to increase her intake even more. A bit cheered, but nonetheless a trifle apprehensive, Em faced the remainder of the day.

After breakfast, she and Jean walked to Pineapplehead, which Em would only be doing twice daily now that she was on maintenance. During the walk she experienced a feeling almost forgotten, hunger. Em had only been hungry a few times when adhering to the original diet, but now she was ravenous! Discussing her plight with Jean, they tried to analyze the situation.

"You are thinking more about food now than ever before, Em. You knew what you'd be eating everyday previously—

94

eating had become second nature. Now that you have choices for breakfast and lunch, you have to think about food before you eat and plan meals the day before. Do you think this has anything to do with it?"

"I do look forward to meals a great deal more than I used to, I suppose, and yes, I do anticipate each meal eagerly. I'm getting hungry now because I'm thinking about all the things I can have for lunch. Tomorrow morning I'll have oatmeal. I haven't had that since my first week on the program. I'll just have to think of something else."

"What will you do with yourself all day, since you won't be walking?"

"Wow, I hadn't thought of that either! I guess I'll sunbathe and write letters. I can start looking through the cookbooks and adapt some recipes, if it doesn't make me hungry. I can't window shop any more. The shopping center is too far away since I've cut my walking down to four miles a day."

"The recipes might make you hungrier Em, but they would help pass the time."

"I'll have to start a project. I brought my sewing machine back and some material. If I buy some patterns, I'll have plenty to keep me busy! Would you drive me to the shopping center for patterns, Jean?"

"Sure will. You need a good project like that, and it will be fun to make new clothes to fit the new you." From then on, it was clear sailing. Em spent many a day inside sewing up a storm, and when she needed a break from zippers and hems, she attacked her cookbooks, adapting tempting recipes to low calorie counts.

Shortly, to Em's delight, the scale again started downhill and a few days later she was able to increase her dinner intake, which turned out to be an experience for everyone. Em found the added bulk almost too much to consume. Her face, everyone observed, turned a strange shade of purple by the end of the meal. She confessed she was so stuffed she could barely breathe.

"It's surprising how much food can be consumed when you watch your calories and use no seasoning," another dieter on maintenance volunteered with an understanding grin. "I experienced the same stuffed feeling, Em. Time for a walk, I think," she suggested. With assistance from all, Em was helped out of her chair and she "waddled" out towards

Pineapplehead. She was still full when she returned, but found the walk had helped pack things down a bit, and she was at least able to talk.

"She's just bragging," Jean chided. "What I would give to be allowed to eat all she ate tonight! I certainly wouldn't put up such a fuss." The next day Em again gained a pound and a half, but expecting the gain, wasn't upset.

Em and Jean remembered to check with the doctors to get the go-ahead for Jean's off-service period with Em. Together they approached the doctors and, after looking at Jean's structured chart, they agreed that the experience would be beneficial to both. Jean assured them that if she found she wasn't losing as well off service, she would return immediately. This announcement was Em's ultimatum—she had high standards to live up to. Jean was reminded that more tests must be taken before she went home and she agreed to make the arrangements.

Once Em's gain from her second increase was lost, she asked the doctors for permission to increase another hundred calories for the remaining few days she would be on the program. Since this would be more than anyone else was allowed, the coordinator gave her a prescription slip giving his permission for her to have free choice of foods. He knew she wouldn't let herself eat more than allowed, and trusted her with this freedom. Em displayed her "prescription" proudly to her friends who were happy for her, but a bit jealous nonetheless.

"What are you eating today?" many would ask her as they inspected her tray. Spotting the extra fruit or salad, they would turn away and sigh.

Em's weight rose again and this time did not go back down quickly. Her doctor cautioned her that each hundred calories she added might take longer for her body to adjust to as she came nearer to her maintenance level. From now on, he emphasized, she should wait at least one week between each increase, even if she starts losing before the week is up. He also suggested increasing by fifty calories a week from this point on, so that her body would not have to adjust to such a drastic change in diet every week. She must be careful and patient during this adjustment period.

* * *

Again, *planning* is the important key in learning to maintain your weight. Em has shown you what to expect. Careful preparation beforehand will permit you to fill your day with activities and structure your thoughts away from food. Constant deliberation of food can be dangerous as you know. Another constructive habit to learn! Eating is *not* our most important objective in life. We simply eat so we can live life to the fullest.

CHAPTER XVII

For two nights the glutton cannot sleep
for thinking,
First on an empty, and next
on a sated stomach.
SA'DI

Em was invited to Washington for a few days during her
last week on service and had made and changed many plans
in the course of preparations during the past two weeks. Her
first decision was to write to her friends telling them that she
would bring all the food she would need except eggs, milk,
and cottage cheese. She would broil chicken breasts and
carry them in a cooler with diet drinks to Washington. They
agreed to this plan, but offered their cooking facilities to her,
saying it would be no problem to cook her meals separately.

"You aren't doing what you're supposed to Em," Jean
scolded her one day. "You aren't supposed to bring your own
food. They'll be glad to skin your chicken for you and omit
the salt. It's not that hard."

"I know, but I just feel I'd be putting them to a lot of trouble."

"Why, Em, they invited you. You won't be putting them out at all. If you were, they wouldn't have invited you in the first place!"

The next evening Em called her friends and told them she'd like to leave the cooking up to them. They were delighted and a bit relieved; Mrs. Berkley would be able to cook everyone's meal together without worrying about warming Em's meal separately.

Em flew to Washington on a Wednesday and the first afternoon was spent avidly discussing behavioral therapy and diet with Mrs. Berkley. The chicken was placed in the oven while they talked, and Mrs. Berkley asked for any special cooking instructions regarding Em's portion. While the chicken cooked they spoke about assertiveness. "Oh dear," Em exclaimed, "I forgot to be assertive enough to ask you to skin my piece." Laughing, they both rushed into the kitchen, took out Em's piece, and skinned it. Em was relieved that Mrs. Berkley hadn't minded at all. They fixed a salad for dinner to accompany the meat and Em made a vinegar spice dressing for everyone. Em remembered all the rules, and by the time everyone else was through, she had eaten only half her chicken and a few mouthfuls of salad, but immediately put down her fork and helped clear the table. That evening Mrs. Berkley took Em to hear a speech at the Junior College outside of town where they joined Mr. Berkley.

The next day Em and her hostess went shopping for special dietetic foods, walked, and generally enjoyed themselves. Mr. Berkley was called out of town on business, so he didn't accompany the two ladies to the opera that night. Every meal was structured and Em remembered all commandments. Mrs. Berkley complimented her on her accomplishments and her determination to stay on the diet.

The next morning Em had breakfast with the family and, since it was raining, Mrs. Berkley drove the children to school. Em, once alone, found her hunger rising and with it, an uncontrollable desire to sneak eat, the old fatal habit. She attacked the cereal boxes and was about to do more damage when she realized this was self-destructive and she must get out of the house. Leaving the dishes until later, she grabbed her coat and started walking. She remembered a friend of hers who had been on the program and lived not far from the Berkleys, so she surprised her with a visit. She discussed her problem with Tania who had left the program a few weeks before. The atmosphere and conversation soon calmed Em and she was ready to go back and clean up the mess she had left.

Returning, Em found the same temptation rising within her, and again grabbed her coat. Her hostess had not returned but had told her she might go to the hairdresser if there was an opening, so Em decided to find her. She did just as Mrs. Berkley was leaving the beauty parlor. Em explained her plight quickly and confessed her "stealing" and apologized. Mrs. Berkley was very understanding, and encouraged Em to keep walking until lunch time if it would help. Em walked the fastest five miles ever and when she returned she was refreshed and had no desire for food.

"It's strange," she told Mrs. Berkley. "I never thought exercise did anything except make you hungrier. I guess that was my lazy obese rationale. I found the more I walked this morning the better I felt, and the less I thought about food."

"What do you suppose brought it on, Em?"

"I don't know. I wasn't upset about anything. As a matter of fact, the past few days have been the happiest in many years. I couldn't ask for any better or nicer friends. Added exercise may have contributed some. We walked a good six or seven miles yesterday and I haven't walked more than four a day for almost two weeks. Then the opera—well, I was pretty tired when we went to bed last night. That's probably what did it."

"I was bushed too last night. I'm glad you could get your eating under control this morning. I too am amazed that walking can work such miracles."

That afternoon Em flew back to her apartment after one of the most enjoyable and most important weekends of her life. She had proven to herself she could get right back on the diet were she unstructured.

* * *

In this chapter we deal with unstructured eating (USE). As Em states, she had an uncontrollable desire to eat, and she did eat. Usually, once USE takes over it mushrooms, and all of our suppressed desires emerge, crying to be satisfied. We are not hungry, but our craving still is in control. How do we stop this?

1. Get away from the situation immediately. True enough, you can't run from your problems, but you can walk—get going!—the faster the better. If for some reason you can't walk, get busy, exercise, do something, anything.

2. Get with a friend, preferably someone who will understand your need. Talk it out: What happened? Why? Where were you? Who were you with? What were you doing? When?

3. Regain your calm. First, take a deep breath. Okay, so you blew it! Admit it. Probably now you're feeling depressed, lonely, upset, hurt, and so on. And next comes all the justifications; how easy it is to rationalize. Of course you can find excuses to eat, all kinds of excuses, and you don't have to look very hard or long. But honestly, will you gain *anything* from feeling sorry for yourself except in pounds and inches? Think about it! And don't think for one minute we don't know what you're going through. We're two old pros, remember?

4. Rebuild your confidence. Begin by erasing your feeling of guilt. We all err. Each day is full of mistakes, but we learn by them and keep going, don't we? This rule applies here also. A habit is learned by repetition, by practicing over and over. Go back to our admonition DON'T TAKE THAT FIRST BITE OF UNSTRUCTURED EATING! and keep going from here.

5. Think of your goal.

6. Begin your dieting again at the next meal, even if it is an hour away. NEVER SKIP A MEAL OR FAST. Believe us, it won't work.

7. Be within calling distance of friends if you feel yourself wanting to backslide. Your strength must be built up again, and a friend's positive reinforcement can do wonders in regaining control.

8. Take a good look at your "before" pictures. Paste them on the refrigerator if necessary.

9. Try on one of your "fatty" outfits and observe how much you have accomplished since beginning your program.

10. Above all, hold your head up and *smile* as you look in the mirror. As your reflection shows, you stand alone. Your objectives, your goals are strictly yours to accomplish. No one can do this for you. Friends can cheer you on, but the desire to succeed comes from within.

Ready? Forward march ... back down the road with us, to a healthier, happier, more beautiful YOU!

CHAPTER XVIII

They perfect nature and are perfected
by experience.
SIR FRANCIS BACON

Jean took the therapist's suggestions for her trip home to heart and started preparations in advance. Realizing she would be spending the first few days traveling, letters were written to everyone with whom she would be staying, telling them her intention to stay structured on the visit, suggesting menus, and giving each an idea of the size portion she would eat. She then busily planned menus for Tom and herself for the remainder of the week when they would be home, writing a grocery list from the menus. Next, she wrote several close friends, telling them when she would be home and that she would like to get together. She wrote of her plans to walk over for the visit since she wouldn't have the car, thereby fitting in needed exercise.

Realizing her family and friends would see a distinct behavioral change, Jean made a list of several points to tell them when all were together. The sooner they began to observe,

103

understand, and adjust to these changes, and the sooner contracts could be put into effect, the easier things would be for all. Her family's education was as important as her own, she felt.

The week before departure, Jean realized she had nothing suitable to wear to Connie's graduation. She had been given two dresses, but neither seemed appropriate for the occasion. This was her first experience at actually trying on clothes and adapting the new styles to her changing figure.

Having no idea what size she wore (having made her own dresses for many years as the stores did not stock her large size), Jean picked out several size eighteen and sixteen dresses that caught her eye. Much to her delight they swallowed her. Surely she couldn't wear a fourteen—it had been years! Bravely marching to the racks with smaller sizes she noticed all the lovely selections from which to choose, much more than on the size eighteen rack. Picking out several she went back to the fitting room, and to her tremendous joy was indeed able to proclaim to the world she could now wear a fourteen. She chose only one dress and was elated at the thought that soon she would be discarding it.

Shoes next, the latest style. Jean had previously had trouble buying shoes because her feet were so wide. But now, slipping into a pair of white heels, she actually felt comfortable. Purse and gloves remained and she would be ready.

During Jean's style show that evening for her landlady and new rooming companion, the three of them selected one of the two dresses given her to wear on the plane, saving her new apparel for the big event.

On the day of departure Jean nervously questioned if her husband would be pleased with her progress. Stepping off the plane she spotted Tom immediately and realized he had looked right past her. Laughing to hide tears of happiness she called to him and waved. Tears streaming down his face, Tom could only say "Momma!" as he grabbed her.

Driving down to her brother Jerry's home the next morning to meet Connie, Tom filled her in on the latest happenings and said he had taken the week off. Jean related some of her experiences and relived a typically structured day. With much to discuss, the trip to Jerry's seemed short. Connie and Sue, Jean's sister-in-law, were sitting on the front lawn wait-

104

ing for them. More tears, bear hugs, kisses, and grins—everyone decided they now needed to diet.

Later Jean asked everyone to sit down as she wanted to explain her changes. Diet drinks in hand, all settled down for a family discussion. Jean told them about the therapy part of the program and how she would adapt her knowledge to the home environment. She would not go back into the old routine of staying home alone night after night because this would lead to withdrawal as in the past. Tom suggested they move closer to his work and rent their house until his retirement in four years, pointing out that she could find work there as well as where they lived now. This sounded good to her and Tom vowed to start looking for an apartment.

She was also learning to think of herself more, she told them, and discussed vanity behavior. "I'll be buying new clothes and trying out new hair styles. I want to go out every once in a while instead of watching television every night."

"You keep the weight off, and I'll see we go out once a week," Tom promised.

With a twinkle in his eye, Jerry acknowledged, "All right, Sis, I remember my promise of a boat trip."

"Fantastic! I'll bring along a bathing suit this time."

Another point she remembered to bring out concerned exercise, "I will need to walk at least two miles every day. How about walking with me after dinner, Tom?"

"Hold on! I have too many speaking engagements at night to stroll around the park with you. Besides, it's too dangerous to be walking alone at night. I'll tell you what—you let me off the hook and I'll buy you a treadmill."

Smiling to herself, Jean realized that they had made a contract with no explanations necessary. "You've got yourself a deal!"

This led to discussing her assertiveness training and she could see favorable nods.

"Seems to me you are being quite assertive just having this discussion!" Jerry commented. They all laughed and Jean realized how right he was. She had changed and, equally as important, her family approved.

All were to have dinner at Jean's niece Sheila's before graduation exercises that night, so they were soon on their way again. Sheila and Connie had planned the meal using

Jean's suggestions, and the meatloaf, salad, and squash, okra, and tomatoes were a big hit. Jean ate a small serving of meatloaf, salad, and iced tea. Washing dishes hurriedly, they all rushed to dress for Connie's big night. The oohs and aahs over Jean's new outfit and figure were almost as rewarding as Connie's bear hugs and Tom's tears.

Graduation exercises were beautiful and, of course, Connie was the prettiest girl there. Tom took rolls of pictures to record the event. Connie had already secured her first job and was now beginning a new life as was Jean.

The next morning Tom and Jean said their goodbyes and headed once again for Jerry's where grilled burgers, a salad, and a vegetable waited. Sue asked many questions about the diet and made many notes on portions and calorie counts. After supper she and Jean paced off an approximate two-mile stretch and Sue vowed she would walk everyday. "Forty minutes isn't too much time each day to spend for your health," Jean encouraged.

The next day Tom and Jerry fished off the dock and promised food for supper. Sue promptly took steaks out of the freezer for grilling. Laughing, the girls planned the menu around steaks, not fish.

"I have baking potatoes, Jean, shall we share one?"

"That's perfect," Jean agreed, showing Sue her portion size of steak. With a salad, the evening meal was planned. The steaks were delicious, topped only by "the five-pounder that got away." Promising a return trip once her goal weight was reached, Jean and Tom headed home. Now comes the true test she thought, realizing she would be cooking for the rest of the week.

Jean shopped strictly from her previously planned menus and her only real problem was getting Tom to the table at mealtime. He was always in the middle of something important. Thank goodness she had remembered those diet drinks. All red and white commandments and newly learned eating habits were strictly adhered to. The scale told her she was continuously losing weight. Having no food scale Jean deduced she was estimating her portions fairly accurately. She managed to walk at least six miles each day at home, and thus kept to her structuring.

The planned visits with friends were delightful. Not one but five and six gathered to see her progress and hear of her experiences. Her assertiveness was not mentioned, although many noticed her changed behavior. As she began her walk back home, she realized most of her friends' lives had changed very little. They still got up each morning, cleaned house, played cards once or twice a week, and that was about all. Most seemed content with this humdrum existence. Surely there was more to life than just this for me, Jean pondered, realizing she wanted something more. Knowing she would have to work again, she started planning her after-work hours. Her hunger for life must be fed from now on with planned activities instead of food.

Packing for the return trip brought Jean pleasure. Going through her closet she found old dresses and shoes. Putting them all in a pile she planned a family burning party upon her next and final trip home. She saved her biggest dress, however, as a constant reminder of what she once wore. Tom reminded her, "In two months you'll have still more to add to the pile!" He was right. During the last two months before reaching goal a person's size changes often and quickly, she had been told by a former dieter.

"Save your pennies," she told Tom. "I'll have a great deal to buy, everything in fact."

With goodbyes said and Jean's promise to take care and finish the job soon, she stepped on the plane. After this very happy week she was anxious to get the next few weeks over with and begin living her new life totally. "How many people are as lucky as I," she wondered, "to have the opportunity to begin again?"

* * *

Both of us returned from our successful trips home having made contracts for future relationships and having shown old friends the "new" persons we were becoming.

Through our individual experiences you have been shown that dieting can continue while traveling or vacationing. Zero in on your objective—you're not vacationing to eat, but to relax, enjoy the companionship of family and friends, absorb your surroundings, take on a new perspective of where you're going in life. Food or nourishment is needed simply to help you reach your life's goals, not hinder your journey toward them.

The next two chapters will answer questions that might arise regarding the practical application of what you have been learning. Now we will show you how to put it all together, how to make it work for you.

CHAPTER XIX

Know how sublime a thing it is
To suffer and be strong.
HENRY WADSWORTH LONGFELLOW

Em and Jean had a happy reunion at the airport and chatted continuously on the way home, each of their own experiences with their families.

That evening they started planning menus for the first week off service: fish, chicken, fish, chicken, and so on for dinners, with steak thrown in once. Breakfasts and lunches were planned separately to accommodate both diets. Jean needed the protein that the three egg whites provided every morning and preferred the low calorie count of the soup to give her as much bulk as possible for her lunch meal. Em was eating oatmeal or dry cereal and from time to time a whole egg for breakfast, and a concoction of tuna fish and cottage cheese for lunch.

Next on the agenda was to decide which of the tempting recipes they would use for their dinners. They decided to try one recipe each meal without repetitions. Jean was eager to learn to cook with herbs and spices, something she had never before attempted. Em, however, had a gourmet for a mother and had learned the tricks of the herb trade when she was seven and eight years old.

Once they decided what recipes to use, they started compiling a grocery list for the week. While doing this their stomachs grumbled and their minds began wandering down unstructured paths. They realized at this rate they were doomed to gain fifty pounds the first week. They had momentarily forgotten the therapist's sage advice: plan menus, write grocery lists, and shop *only* on full stomachs. To make certain of success they waited until after dinner to tackle the problem again. They found their revised list structured and no sounds coming from their stomachs. They tackled the supermarket in the same manner and found the "whistles and hums" practically inaudible. Buying proportionately cut their food bill immensely and no leftovers remained to add temptation. A pocket calorie counter became their constant companion during meal planning and grocery shopping and helped them stay away from any tempting goodies despite the fact that they paid the grocery bill by check instead of bringing just enough cash to cover the food cost as their therapist had suggested. The cupboards remained bare of unstructured food. Menus were changed at the supermarket occasionally when the prices were too high or fresh vegetables were not available. Substitutions were made for some items and others were eliminated altogether. The tight budget and anticipation of extra money for their new wardrobes were great incentives to buy wisely from their structured list.

They soon realized Em's kitchen was too small for both, so an agreement was made that Em would cook and Jean became chief bottlewasher. This contract turned out to be excellent, as Jean was still walking twelve to fourteen miles each day. Keeping her day structured left little time to plan and prepare meals.

Em, on the other hand, was busy during a certain part of the day with cooking, adapting and inventing new recipes, and writing each on three by five cards with calorie counts per portion to boot for both recipe boxes. After each new invention was tried, an original name after events or thoughts that cropped up during the day and a comment would be written on the top line of the recipe card: good, fair, scrumptious, out of this world, omega, the living end.

The kitchen was always highly organized and clean. "A place for everything and everything in its place" became the household motto. Em found little time to be bored now which was a relief after the trials she had been through the previous week with trying to find things to do.

After two weeks off the program, a beautifully structured routine was worked out. Jean was still losing steadily and Em's calorie count had finally begun mounting again. She had endured a rough three weeks adjusting to her increase, but after that there seemed to be much less problem. The scale did what was expected: go up a few pounds the first day or two, level off, and then come down again. But, as all good things must come to an end, they found their routine one day fractured.

While taking their usual after dinner walk to Pineapplehead (Em joined Jean on the two-miler after breakfasts and dinner), Jean tripped up a flight of stairs, fracturing one wrist bone and crushing another. About midnight, after five hours in the Emergency Room, Em drove her home. Both collapsed in their beds.

At breakfast the next morning they faced the changes that would have to be made. Em found herself doing all the kitchen chores as Jean's left arm was in a cast from fingers to just below her shoulder. Em was even called on to tie Jean's shoes and wash her right arm. Too tired to make any new contracts that day, they both rested and spent the day waiting for the doctor to examine Jean's cast to make sure all was right. He spent what seemed like thirty seconds with her after she waited two hours, and told her to report back in a week for X-rays and another check, one for her arm and another from her bank. That night they had "Emergency Room Fish" for dinner, the description of which was "Smashing."

The next morning Em picked Jean up and drove to the dining room for their early morning before-breakfast weigh-in. Much to their astonishment Jean had gained only one-half pound, cast and all. "Surely this thing weighs more than that! It feels like I'm carrying around a ton."

After breakfast Jean made preparations for the morning two-miler and asked Em to tie her shoes. "You're not going anywhere but to lie down. You couldn't make it around the block, and you plan to walk to Pineapplehead?"

"Then I've got to cut down my eating or I'll gain more weight."

Em's patience with this nonsense had about reached the end and it showed in her next comment: "You have to eat to keep up your strength and heal your arm. Now go lie down."

By this time Jean was beginning to realize Em was right, but not quite willing to admit how weak she was feeling. "Talk about aggressive behavior!" she retorted.

"This is a perfect example of positive assertiveness and you know it, now GIT!"

Jean got, and slept three hours until noon. During lunch Em watched her nearly fall asleep in her soup and put her foot down once again as she started to take her bowl into the kitchen. "Stop it," Em demanded. "I'm not going to put up with your stubbornness. I am doing all the work around here from now on and in return I want just a little cooperation from you. You will now go into the bedroom and lie down while I wash dishes. When you wake up we will have supper and I will then take you home and you will go right to bed. I will pick you up in the morning. Period. Case closed." Jean got the message this time, fumbled her way to the bed, and was once again instantly in a deep sleep.

In the peace and quiet Em managed to regain her composure by keeping busy: cleaning up the kitchen, pouring through cookbooks, and fixing the evening meal. Jean woke just before supper. After eating a delicious meal she was again exhausted and furious with herself for being so. There were no arguments this time when they headed for the car.

The next morning Jean was sensible enough to know she needed her rest. She was puzzled about this need though and talked about it with Em.

"I can't understand it, Em," she said. "I've always been able to bounce right back after my several operations. The doctors have always been amazed at my speedy recoveries. You wouldn't think this arm would cause me so much trouble. I can't help feeling awful. I've never been helpless before or waited on this much. I feel guilty not walking at least eight miles a day. I haven't even done two in the past two days."

"I know exactly how you feel, Jean, because I'm the same way, and so is my father. Our kind makes the world's worst patient. But I also can see how tired you are, and besides you're adhering strictly to your diet. How can you expect your body to cope with your arm on such a small intake? So please, do what I tell you and get your rest. The more resting you do now, the less days you'll feel this bad, and the sooner you'll be able to walk those eight miles again."

"It hadn't occurred to me that the diet would make the difference but I guess you're right. I'll tell you what: you're doing all the kitchen work, so I'll treat you to a dinner out once a week. Plus, as you already know, you have free use of my car whenever you need it. Okay?"

Em smiled at her for the first time since the accident. It was an excellent contract, Em was greatly relieved, and the tension lifted. She returned to being her normal self even though she still had to occasionally remind the bucking Jean of her limitations.

* * *

There are several things to bring to your attention in this chapter. First, you *can* cook two different meals simultaneously. If your spouse were put on a low-cholesterol or salt-free diet, you would adjust, wouldn't you? Are your needs any less important? A little preplanning and a few extra minutes will solve your problems.

Now, a caution about supermarkets. Shopping for food immediately after a meal can be as dangerous for some as shopping when hungry for others. So find a time of day at which you are most comfortable and least tempted around food to do your shopping. Because each person is different and has different schedules, everyone will have a best time to shop. Find it, and use it!

Second, as Jean learned, cooking with herbs and spices is fun. We do caution you, however, to begin with a very small amount and work up since too much can ruin a good meal. The joy of using different flavorings is that, besides adding taste to foods, most are non-caloric. This brings us to another constructive habit that must be formed: READ THE LABELS. Not all "Diet" foods are low in calories. The word "Diet" generally means that the food has been processed in

113

a different way than most, i.e., low in cholesterol, low in sodium, etc. Low-cholesterol food is not necessarily low-calorie. Some spices have added salt in them. Some foods are packaged in water, some in syrup, some items are breaded. Reading the labels before buying will save money and unneeded frustration.

Third, write your favorite recipes down. You may wish to add to or subtract from the original according to your particular taste. Besides, it is much easier to find a three-by-five card from a box as opposed to thumbing through several cookbooks filled with luscious, unstructured, and tempting photographs.

To regain composure, you don't necessarily have to work around food as Em did in this case. Some find needlepoint, knitting, crewel work, or sewing soothing. Others find carpentry, painting, designing, decorating, or gardening relaxing. Usually your favorite hobby is one of the most calming for you. If you don't have one, start one. This can be a perfect outlet for your pent-up emotions, and you will find joyous relaxation when you involve yourself in it. There are many ways to rationalize away your diet. It is so convenient to blame circumstance at times as Jean could have done. So keep your guard up—keep smiling at the "new" reflection you are building.

CHAPTER XX

Good,
the more communicated,
more abundant grows.
JOHN MILTON

The only other tension they both experienced during those
few days after the accident was Em's irritability. She did not
understand why she had suddenly become so touchy, and all
Jean knew was that when Em snapped, it was time to leave
her alone. Cautious, wanting to keep their relationship on an
even keel, Jean became quite sensitive to the effect her dis-
ability was having on Em's patience.

A routine had been established of weighing in every
morning before breakfast. Jean was still losing, though a bit
more slowly, and both were thrilled that, despite the fact she
had not gained the strength back to do much walking, she
was still losing. They discussed this at breakfast one
morning.

"I can't figure out how I could still be losing, Em. I haven't done anything but eat, sleep, and walk a few times around the block since I broke this darned arm."

"Don't ask questions, Jean, your body might get the idea and stop! Just be grateful. Besides, your protein must be going somewhere since you're always tired."

"That's true. I guess the energy I'd normally be expending walking is being used to heal my arm."

Jean had been noticing that although weight and diet were still the main topics of conversation, Em, since beginning maintenance, had stopped discussing her own weight. She also noticed that although she was regaining strength, Em still seemed depressed. At weigh-in one morning Jean asked her how her weight was doing.

Em shrugged, "Okay."

"Well, what do you weigh now? You look depressed."

"I'm the same as always since maintenance, 125."

"That's great!" Jean exclaimed, trying to put some enthusiasm into the conversation.

"I suppose so. How did you do today?"

"I lost a half. What's wrong, Em? What's bothering you?"

"Nothing, I'll be okay." Em's face only got longer. After a long silence she decided to tell all. "I know it's stupid to feel this way, but for some reason I'm jealous of your weight loss. I'm not losing any more and for so long the scale was my biggest reward. You are still being rewarded, but I'll never be able to have that feeling again unless I gain first."

"Is this why you have been depressed these past few days?" Jean asked, and Em nodded.

"Well, it will help me, and I think you too, if we analyze this, as I'll be going through the same thing soon. Would you mind discussing it, Em?"

"I'd like to, Jean, because I've noticed I haven't been able to control my temper lately, and since you're the person closest to me, you get the brunt of my anger, even though you haven't done anything to deserve it."

"You're going to have to learn to control your temper, Em, because other people who don't know you as well as I do might take offense when you are edgy. I understand you, so I realize your frustrations are not because of me. You'll have to deal with your frustrations in some other way. If you talk

116

about them they won't be trapped inside you and this may help relieve the tension, like a pressure cooker."

"Yes, I can see how communication would be very important. It also means I must bring everything out into the open. *Honesty* is the most vital factor. This isn't always easy."

"The door to communication closes the moment we stop being honest with each other and ourselves, Em. There is no way to help someone who keeps even one fact hidden. If you and I can keep this door open it will be a great help to both of us. Let's start with your problem. Are you tempted to cut your calories to get the reward from the scale?"

"I have been underestimating my calories because of it. When I left the program I was 135. I've lost ten pounds since then. Most medical charts say with my height I should weigh about 132."

"You'll have to stop losing then, Em. You'll get sick if you go any lower. Can you find another reward to take the place of the scale?"

"Facing the scale every day is one habit I never want to break. Walking is another. If I get out of those two habits, I'll have nothing to stop me from gaining. I could fall right back to my old habits and bad routine again, ending up right back where I started."

"What else do you do every day, then, besides weigh and walk?"

Em chuckled. "Eat!" she commented.

"All right," replied Jean with a twinkle in her eyes. "What reward can you establish there?"

"Well, I'll be getting a slow cooker and blender soon. I can try new recipes. I could buy cookbooks, but not every day. My scale reward is daily. I can't afford to buy something new every day."

"Have you been walking more than your four miles a day?"

"No. I realize I have to keep my mileage down."

Jean thought about all this as they walked back to the apartment in silence. "Maybe this is what the doctors mean when they say to put less emphasis on the scale so when we get to maintenance this absence of reward doesn't throw us."

"In other words then, the scale should be my guide, not

my reward. If I gain weight one day, I can look back in my diary at what I ate the day before and find out why I gained. It's to be my red light. Without it I might not catch my gain until it's too late and I'm falling down that mountain with no way to stop until I hit rock bottom again."

"And it should also be your red light for weight loss, Em. If you go below 125 you should increase your calories."

"But I'm eating so much! You know how full my plate is every night. By the way, does my plate full of food bother you?"

Jean smiled. "Watching you eat is good therapy for me. Tom will be eating that much and more when I go home and I'll have to live with it. This is a good experience for me. But to get back to your food, Em, you're eating a great deal of low-calorie food. If you started using butter and other supplements in your cooking you'd be adding calories without bulk. You'd have to watch out for sodium, though."

"No, I have increased my sodium to the normal level, so I can eat prepared foods now. I just stay away from adding any salt at the table."

"That's great. All I've heard you talk about lately is how you'd like an English muffin. If you've increased your salt count, you can have it. Why don't you look in the calorie counter and see how many calories an English muffin and a tablespoon of butter are? But so help me, if you bring crunchy peanut butter into the house, I'll shoot you!"

Brightening, her face taking on an eager expression, Em said, "That's a great idea. I could freeze the extra muffins so I wouldn't be tempted to eat them all at once. Peanut butter is out though, I could never stop at a tablespoonful and I can't freeze that. At least I wouldn't be as tempted by plain butter." Em grabbed her calorie counter when they reached her apartment and found she'd be able to eat a muffin with one tablespoon of butter for breakfast with an egg and coffee. "A perfect breakfast, Jean . . . ," she shouted, her spirits soaring. The door was open and Em happily spent the rest of the morning with her head buried in her calorie counter. As long as she watched her calories, she would have no problems.

Jean, returning from her before-lunch walk around the block, found Em surrounded by cookbooks and the calorie counter and began worrying about her own structured eating. "Em, I think it's time for some more honest communication.

I've told the doctors that if I don't lose as well off the program as I did on service, I'll go back to eating there."

"I've been doing all I can, Jean, to keep your diet intact, and everything I cook has been as structured as I can make it. If you want, I'll cut out all the herbs and spices and give you the food exactly as they prepare it in the cafeteria. I need your companionship, and I'll do anything you want to your food to help you lose weight."

"Do herbs and spices add calories or sodium, then?"

"No, not in moderation. A moderate amount of them make no difference at all. But if it will make you feel better, I'll stop using them on your food."

"Heaven forbid! I'm enjoying it. I'm doing fine so far. Don't worry, I'll let you know if any changes have to be made. I guess the idea of your eating a toasted cheese sandwich got to me. That with a bowl of chili really would hit the spot." They both laughed when they added up those calories.

"I think it will be a few years before I can even dream of eating that," Em sighed.

"Maybe when I reach maintenance I can have an English muffin, too," Jean said dreamily.

"You won't be able to eat them, Jean. The doctors have said you must remain salt-poor for the rest of your life, and English muffins do have sodium."

"Oh, heck! Well, at least I know my limitations and can start preparing and planning now. Some foods are just going to be a No-No for me. I'll have to remember to read the ingredients on all the packages of food carefully before I buy anything. It never occurred to me that English muffins would have salt.

"Won't you be glad, Em, when you find your maintenance level so you won't have the guess work any more? I'm anxious to get on maintenance to find mine. Then, if I should go visiting for a weekend, knowing that I have stayed at my calorie level, I won't have to bother jumping on the scale."

"For me it will be different. I'm going to depend on the scale every morning to tell me whether I ate enough or too much the previous day. Right now, I seem to be always hungry because I'm always thinking about what I can add to the next meal. My life is still based around food, but in a different way than four or five months ago. Then I ate all the time. Now I *think* about eating all the time."

Both laughed, realizing how true this was. "We all think about food when we're on a diet, I guess, because that is where our main thrust at the moment lies. Thinking about it doesn't make me hungry, though. As a matter of fact, after four months of dieting I find myself satisfied with these smaller portions, and for the first time in years, I can actually tell when I'm full."

"I used to feel full too, amazingly enough, but once I was allowed more my hunger increased. I hope that doesn't happen to you."

"I hope not, Em. I've decided not to add bulk right away. I'll start by adding the supplements so I won't get used to more quantity. My maintenance level will probably be very low anyway."

"You can't tell, Jean, so there's no need worrying about it yet. I didn't think I'd get higher than a daily 800 calories, but my metabolism or something must have changed, because I'm eating 1250 now and still losing."

"Well, I certainly hope you're right. In any case, we'll have to have some activities planned for when we do reach maintenance, since we won't be spending as much time thinking of food. Your free time will be well taken care of at college, I imagine, both during the day and after dinner. I'll be working every day, but I have never had a social life before. I'll have to find ways to get out of the house. Tom has agreed to take me out at least once a week. Maybe a good idea would be not to have a television in our new apartment. My evening walk will take time and I'm determined to keep that habit. When I came on the program the doctors said they were willing to bet me that when I reached my goal, walking two miles every day would be the one thing I wouldn't do. At least you won't have to worry about walking at college; you'll probably find yourself over-walking and having to increase your calories."

"What are you going to do at night, Jean?"

"I don't know. I'll have to wait until I go home."

"No, that's exactly what we have to plan for now. Preparation is the key, remember?"

"Well, my problem is I don't know when Tom will have a speaking engagement. Sometimes I'll be able to go with him, and sometimes I won't."

"But you have to plan some alternatives, Jean, so you don't end up with spare time. That only leads back to where you were before."

"Maybe I can start bowling again. I could go back to my piano and organ playing."

"You should write contacts in your new home town and make plans."

"But I don't know anyone there, Em. I'll have to make a whole new set of friends. Practicing the organ for church will take some time, anyway."

"But Jean, you have to start getting involved with other people. That was the therapist's comment when you first entered the program, remember?"

"You're right. I can get involved with church work and meet people there. My new home town has a civic center, too. I'll look into that. Maybe some new acquaintances will go to the football games with me if Tom won't. I'm an avid sports fan."

"There you go! You see, there are lots of things you could do if you take the time to look for them. You've been living for too long waiting for others to call you. Now you must start taking the initiative and live for yourself. Only when you show that you have confidence in and respect for yourself will others have respect for you and start wanting to be with you."

"The only thing I dread is Tom showing me off to all his friends. I'm proud of my accomplishments, and I want people to accept me the way I will be—not because I look better than I did before. I want to forget the past and start fresh. I have changed not only physically, but mentally, and because this isn't outwardly visible, people who compare me to the way I was will assume I'm the same person. Hopefully, people will soon see the complete new me."

"Jean, if you want to start completely new, you're going to have to abandon this silly idea of yours that you're going to save money by taking in some of the clothes you are wearing now. I'm going to tell you exactly what my parents told me— you deserve a whole new wardrobe. After all the work you've put into this 'new person' you must throw away all your old clothes, leaving no remembrances of your past. If you want others to stop comparing the old to the new you, you must do

121

the same. Besides, it's too easy to take something in now and let the seams out later. If you can't take anything out, you'll decrease the temptation to gain even five pounds, because you won't have anything that fits."

"All right Em, you'd better heed your own advice. Since you are at goal, I suggest we take a shopping trip this afternoon to buy you some clothes for college, something nice that you can be proud to wear. You won't be wearing your new dresses to class. Besides, didn't your father say you ought to buy everything you need here since there are no department stores near your home? Anyway, this will give me an opportunity to see what styles I'll soon be wearing. I might even try on a dress or two to see what size I am now. Maybe I can fit into a twelve. I have only fifteen more pounds to go, so I might be able to judge what size I'll be at goal."

"You're no twelve, Jean, at most you're a ten. That graduation dress looks like a potato sack now. Besides, the last twenty pounds always makes the most difference in inches."

After lunch they were on their way. Em tried on many pairs of slacks, running out of the dressing room to model each one. She decided on a few and selected coordinating tops to compliment her choices. Jean began to tire, so they decided to find a place to relax with a cup of coffee.

Over coffee Jean asked Em about her plans for her social life at college. "Em, how are you going to cope with your emotional life? No one knows what you've been doing on your leave of absence and the oohs and aahs won't last more than a couple of days. Then your old friends will discover you've changed emotionally as well. You may even find you can't get along with some of your old friends any more, especially if they aren't willing to accept the new you."

"That's true . . . I *may* find myself with a whole new set of friends," replied Em thoughtfully. "One thing for sure, I won't go back to being a doormat for anyone now or I'll be asking for trouble. I'll have to make many contracts with friends."

"You know, Em, this is going to take patience on our part too. We can't expect our friends to accept the new us over night; patience and assertiveness must be developed. We better start practicing how to be honest and open in an assertive way with those back home."

"Right! You and I began our friendship candidly and have worked out our problems. We don't hide our feelings from each other. But at college it's different. Naturally, my friends will assume our old relationship—the bottles of rum, and all." Thoughtfully the two pondered this new discovery.

"Em, maybe you could lay some groundwork through your correspondence. You still have a couple of months before school starts. Something else we're going to have to face, too, is that some will not like our changes."

"On the other hand, Jean, we also will be acquiring new friends, and they won't know the old us. And this new relationship will be built on openness and honesty, as ours has been."

"I guess the secret here is not to dwell on the past. If our friendship is rejected by some, we must learn to accept this and cultivate new ones."

"Here is where our self-confidence can not waiver. What is best for us must come first. Besides Jean, no one really likes a doormat. No one really cares for a person of whom they can take advantage."

"Yes, I can see your point. You'll be going back to a different situation than before, Em. Instead of a dorm, you'll be living off campus with other students. You'll have a roommate who knew the old you and has no idea you're changing. How are you going to cope with your eating habits? When I was in college, we ate hamburgers and french fries after studying those long hours."

"I'll have the kitchen to myself since the others will be eating in the college cafeteria. My roommate doesn't know I've been on a diet and my changes will force our relationship to change, I know. Complete openness and honesty with each other will have to be the first and most important factor in our new relationship. I'll have to sit everyone in the house down when I get there and make contracts about my eating, just as you did with your family. There will be times when I'll want to eat with them, and I'll depend on the scale every day to tell me how I'm doing and how I should structure my eating the next day. They will have to avoid tempting me, though."

"Em, you're bound to have leftovers since you'll be cooking for just yourself. How will you handle them?"

"I've found I am much less tempted to nibble frozen leftovers, so I think I'll freeze them in separate packages proportionately."

"Great idea! You can put on the outside of the carton how much it contains. That's a fabulous idea for me too. I can freeze Tom's leftovers as well, that way keeping my fingers out of forbidden food."

"The only leftovers I'll keep in the refrigerator will be the ones I'll use right away.

"I had better buy an extra set of measuring cups, too, so I won't have any excuse for not being accurate. I've found I am sometimes too lazy to wash the measuring cups, leading me to guess at portion size. One thing I am sure to do, though, is measure our meat portion. One-half ounce of meat really makes a difference calorie-wise. The more I control my portions too, Jean, the less leftovers I'll have."

Coffee finished, the two shoppers headed for the dress department. Jean looked at the size twelve rack and found three dresses she wanted to try on.

"Where do I go to try these on, Em?"

"Let me see those—size twelve? Jean, you're crazy. Take those back and look at the tens. And you can forget the pleated skirts too, and that dark blue. You don't need those camouflages anymore; you can wear anything you want."

Both looked at the size tens and found several to try on. While Jean wasn't looking, Em slipped a size seven in the group.

In the dressing room Em helped Jean into the size seven. "Where did you find this?" Jean asked, admiring the bright colors and soft line. Finding her cast a bit clumsy for trying on clothes she was grateful for Em's assistance—first over the cast, then the head, then the other arm, and zip. Surely there was an easier way! Both realized only sleeveless dresses could be tried on.

"Look Em, it's perfect. I can wear a ten!"

"I have a confession to make, Jean," Em said beaming at her. "This is a size seven!"

"No way, Em." Showing Em the tag Jean became momentarily speechless. "Good heavens!" she exclaimed, her face radiant. "Connie wears size nine. Em, I can't remember ever wearing this size before."

"Do you realize this means you'll be in sizes five and six when you reach goal in a few weeks?"

"Let's look at the fives and sixes, Em. I'm so excited."

Looking at the lower size rack they found very few from which to choose. "This is amazing," Jean exclaimed. "When I started this diet no store in my town carried my large size and now that I'll be in fives and sixes I can't find any either. All of these are too short for me. I've gone from one extreme to the other."

"Try this six on, Jean. It's so pretty, and the colors would be perfect with your black hair." Em had produced a white dress with an embroidered bodice in green, yellow, red, and black. "You may not be able to fit into it now, but we'll be able to see if you can in a few weeks."

Jean tried it on and Em zipped it up. "It's snug, but should be perfect when I reach goal. I'll have to buy earrings and shoes to match. It's just beautiful."

They bought the dress plus two others, one size seven and one size five for later. Jean was in seventh heaven and planned future shopping trips for accessories.

It was about time for supper and both were tired. They talked avidly about their new purchases and planned glorious parties around them. The two laughed and chatted, wondering which outfit their knights on white chargers would approve of most highly.

"When Tom comes on his mighty steed, Jean, you'd really look like a queen in that white dress. But you'll have to sit sidesaddle," Em teased. "I've been more practical. I can jump up behind my knight in my white pants and won't have to worry about being ladylike."

They decided to eat out for dinner, choosing steak from the menu.

"I hope you realize, Em, you're going to have to help me with this steak. I certainly don't want to gain any weight now, and you haven't eaten your full allotment today."

"Glad to be of service, Madam!"

"I'm anxious to try out that slow cooker you're getting, Em. I hope there's a recipe book with it."

"That's going to be great fun to try. My mother has one she seldom uses, and I think hers has a recipe book. If mine doesn't, I'll just snitch hers when I go home."

"Will we be able to adapt recipes to it?"

"Anything cooks in the slow cooker. The great thing about it is that you can throw everything in it in the morning, turn it on, and when you're ready for the evening meal, dinner is ready for you."

"That sounds fabulous."

"The only thing I wouldn't want to put in a slow cooker is a good steak like this," Em commented as she ate half of Jean's.

Em returned to her apartment that evening to find her blender and cooker, complete with recipe book. The next morning their weekly menus and grocery list were constructed around the use of the new appliances.

They started grocery shopping later than usual because of all the extra planning, and returned to the apartment an hour after their hunger alarm clocks had sounded. Em was very irritable and Jean stayed out of her way. Em slopped the soup all over the table and forgot utensils and napkins in her hurry. Everything went wrong until she managed to absorb some nourishment. After a few bites she calmed down a bit.

"Wow! That will teach us never to shop so late again. I thought I was going to die of starvation," Jean commented once the storm passed.

"You're so right. I'm really sorry I snapped at you, but when I'm that hungry, I just can't do anything right. I was shaking, I was so famished."

"It's a good thing we had our grocery list and each other, or we would have bought out the whole store. Before I forget, let me pay you my half. I have the cash here now."

"I'd rather you pay me by check, Jean. Then I won't have to worry about loose change, and I'll have to deposit it into my account."

"I always carry cash with me. It doesn't bother me in the least. But I'll write you a check if you prefer. It seems to me that since you're almost at your maintenance level, you'd have that problem under control. Sooner or later you're going to have to work that problem out, Em."

"How true, Jean, but for now I just don't want to invite temptation. Since my will power is still weak, I must control my environment carefully."

That afternoon a friend of theirs from the program called. "My wife is returning home after her visit and I must get all these unstructured leftovers out of my apartment. Could you use them?"

"We'll be right over, Erv, thanks," Em told him. "We accept charity here," she laughed.

Erv gave them eggs, strawberries, salad materials, all of which could be used easily. He also gave them two boxes of crackers, which fast proved to be Em's downfall.

"Jean, I can't stand it any longer," Em confided at dinner one night. "I haven't told you this before, but I'm having a lot of trouble with leftovers. You always leave something on your plate at dinner, and when I clear the table I put them in my human garbage disposal. I can't control the urge. It's not hurting my weight, but it's a very lethal habit. Lately I've been uncontrollably tempted to eat those crackers Erv gave us."

"Oh wow, Em. That's awful. I'm going to have to face that, too. Plate cleaning was one of my worst habits. Maybe we can find a solution. First of all though, we must throw out the crackers, not here but downstairs in the garbage can."

"Would you watch me while I do it? I'm really afraid I'll sneak one if someone isn't there to watch me."

"All right, but I'm not going to watch you every time you take the plates into the kitchen. If you are honest with yourself you won't eat the scraps."

"What do you mean? I don't understand."

"If you know that I know your problem, Em, you won't be tempted to eat the scraps, knowing you'll have to account to me. If you don't eat them, I'll be proud of you and you'll be pleased with yourself."

"So, I really wouldn't have to tell you because you'd know anyway by my face, if I look happy or guilty."

"That's right, and just the idea that you might have to account for what you did may help keep you structured. But more important, Em, we aren't going to have each other's support once we leave here and begin our new life. In these few remaining weeks we must concentrate on strengthening our desire to remain structured. It's not all going to be roses, therefore we must always keep our goal foremost in our minds. It's up to us and only us to maintain our diet the rest of our lives. Maybe a good idea to help us through this situation would be to clear the table just as soon as we've stopped eating so we don't have to sit here looking at our scraps."

"Sometimes we won't be able to clean our plates right

away, Jean. I guess this is where portion control comes in. The key to avoiding leftovers then is to plan not to have any. I never want to go back to the sneak eating habit. What I eat I want to eat in front of everyone. I'll have to be as honest with everyone as you and I are with each other."

"Would it help if I leave a bite on my plate every night so that you can get used to this and overcome your bad habits?"

"I guess that would be a good idea. When I was home I noticed everyone left something on their plates, no matter how much or little they had been served. I'm going to have to learn to control myself."

"Let's start right now. We should solve these problems while we're here. I'm finished—take my plate out and throw the leftovers away."

Em did and came back beaming triumphantly. "I did it, Jean! And now I know that since I did it once, I can do it again." The more she practiced the easier her new habit became, and soon she felt completely at ease when clearing the table.

A few more weeks passed by and Em was maintaining her weight on 1400 calories per day. The scale neither went up or down and Em relaxed. "It's strange, Jean," she remarked one day. "I always thought I'd be unhappy to find my maintenance level because that would mean I wouldn't be able to eat any more. But I feel so much more at ease now that I know how much I can eat. I can get used to this level and start judging my portions by sight instead of counting every calorie. It's really a relief."

"You know, like me, you'll never be able to eat some foods though, Em. Doesn't that depress you a bit?"

"Well, I guess I could start feeling sorry for myself, say it isn't fair that some people can eat all they want of everything, but this sort of rationalizing must not ever begin. A diabetic must adhere strictly to his prescribed diet; an alcoholic can have no alcohol. They cannot dodge the issue, and neither can we. Period. Case closed!"

Laughing, the two friends remembered Em using these same words to stress another point—Jean's need of rest to mend her fractured wrist. Jean left for her afternoon walk and Em scheduled an appointment to go through her check-out behavioral tests for the therapist.

"Hey Jean, wait up," shouted Sharon. Always glad to have company, Jean was happy to see another dieter friend. "You know, you really do look good," complimented Sharon, "not only weightwise, but your color has returned since you broke your wrist. Are you still staying on your diet and nursing that arm too?"

"Oh yes," Jean answered smiling. "I don't have the energy to do as much walking as I did though. The doctors have asked me about my diet this past week and they seem pleased I'm eating a well-balanced one. Their only comment was to increase my protein some."

"Are you still losing as much as you normally did?"

"No, my losing pattern has slowed down some, but then I'm not walking as much as I used to either. Once I get my full strength back and start on my regular twelve- to fourteen-mile routine again, I'll lose more. Didn't we have a lecture one time that brought out the fact that excess body fat is from our lack of activity to use up what we take in?"

"Right, I remember that one. Our food intake and our energy output must be in balance to keep our weight stable."

"Well, I guess I'm pretty well-balanced, because I'm not losing much. But right now my arm is the most important thing, I think."

Jean returned from her walk and found Em back from her tests. "How did check-out go?"

"Believe it or not, I took the same tests I did when we came on the program. Remember those questions about our feelings, our attitudes about people, food, situations, and all? It really was amazing, Jean, because they made me see how much I have changed. My feelings about everything then were entirely different than they are now!"

"What changes have you made?"

"Well, when I took the tests before, I put down the answers I *thought* were right. For instance, if the question was about my behavior in a certain situation, I put down the way I thought I should behave. But this time my answers to the same situations were honest and they turned out to be the same answers I thought were right five months ago.

"When I arrived, I was a non-assertive person. I learned to be assertive by practice these past months and the tests showed that not only has my outward behavior changed, but

129

also my attitudes. I have begun to think assertively and believe in what I say and do."

"Then what you're saying Em, is that you were ready for this change when you first came on the program."

"Yes, I was desperate. I was open for any suggestions that might help and I was willing to try any professional advice, medical and emotional, that might put me on the right track. I can honestly say that had I not been completely open for help and willing to accept any advice without question, I would never have made progress or gained the confidence I now have."

"It's exactly the same for me," Jean reflected. "I was ready to accept any medical advice to lose weight. I wanted and needed medical supervision. But when I arrived here I didn't know anything about behavioral therapy. I didn't know what it was and I didn't see any relationship between my emotions and dieting then. After five months on this program, however, I realize now that by having opened myself to the behavioral part as well, I have discovered this therapy is the base for all successful dieting and will also be the determining factor for my successful weight control in the future."

"This therapy we will constantly be applying is our *own* behavior though, Jean, not just behavior in general. The first thing we learned was to think of ourselves before anything else, and this was the first step in our changing process."

"In other words, Em, we had to be ready to change first—then, by putting ourselves first, our rehabilitation began."

"By the same token, the first thing our family and friends must accept is that we *have* put ourselves first emotionally and physically. By showing them this they should realize that we are now controlling our own lives. Only when we are in control of ourselves will we find true happiness and peace of mind."

"But the same problems will still be at home, Em, when we go back."

"Yes, but we have our knowledge and assertiveness now to help us solve those problems. How to tear down the walls we have previously built is what we must discover."

"I see," commented Jean, beginning to appreciate the total picture. "We'll have to tear those walls down brick by brick with our assertiveness and by communicating openly and honestly with everyone."

"What do you mean 'brick by brick'?"

"Well Em, those walls or problems have been built and reinforced slowly throughout our life. We can't expect to go home and have everyone instantly agree to forget everything in the past and start fresh. We have to work out each detail slowly and carefully and iron out one wrinkle at a time, or take one brick off the wall at a time. The only way we can do this is by putting our own feelings foremost and communicating these feelings no matter how small, openly, honestly, and assertively, establishing a firm foundation for sound contracts. And then our loved ones will be able to share completely and truthfully with us."

"Well, you should let some of the little details go by, Jean, to keep your mind focused on the main wall."

"The small details made the foundation though, Em. This is where complete honesty comes in. Nothing can be hidden any more. You're physically ready to go home. Are you also ready to face those bricks?"

"Yes, Jean, I am. I ran away from that wall and hit rock bottom. Now I have learned to face those bricks and how to start tearing them down to build a firmer, stronger foundation."

"Rock bottom again, Em, but this time we have all the necessary building material within us. Just think—if we take each brick of that wall off carefully, we can use those same bricks to build more solid contracts for a new and better life."

* * *

We must emphasize very strongly that reaching goal does *not* mean you are through. You never will be. You are simply ready for the last important step. Your doctor will structure for you a balanced daily eating program according to your personal needs and desires when you are ready for maintenance. And, because finding your maintenance level can take several weeks, we caution you to go slowly, increasing your calorie intake by small amounts as Em did. You must give your body time to adjust and start functioning at the new food intake level. You didn't gain all of your excess baggage overnight and you haven't lost it overnight.

131

May we bring out again as we did in this last chapter and in the Introduction that reaching goal does *not* mean you will live happily ever after. Problems will always be present—every rose bush has its thorns. We hope that you have already discovered that these difficulties can be met with the clearer perception that honesty and openness allow. We no longer need to hide within our obesity. We are free of this heavy burden for today. The tendency toward overweight, however, is ever-present. As long as we are willing to admit we are obese, the first and main difficulty in controlling our environment has been conquered.

As you must by now be aware, this program is a self-centered one. No one opened our mouths and stuffed the food in and, as you have learned, no one can do the dieting for you. No problems that crop up, however large or small, must keep us from our goal. Yes, at times we *will* be lonely, we will be depressed and hurt. This is part of life. We have learned ways to overcome these situations. The question we forever ask is, "What is best for me?"

Now that we are free of our bulges and spare tires, we find we can also discard some of the constant concern so necessary for successful dieting. As we have disposed of some of "us" we have room to take on an added dimension. Research has revealed that approximately fifty percent of the American population is overweight. With complete confidence in our own ability to admit our limitations and to successfully structure our daily lives, we are now joyfully in a position to tell the world, to extend our good fortune to others, to share.

How? There are several ways. Writing a book as we have is one. More important though, is being a shining, living example. Let others see the beauty of the world through your rebirth. Sharing will also help combat loneliness, depression, and boredom. As Robert Morell so aptly phrased it, "The first great gift we can bestow on others is a good example."

We have shown you through these pages how to build a better you. We can lead you no further. The application for continued success must come from within each one of us. We have learned to take each day at a time. Today we are healthier, happier, more beautiful people within. And, with continued determination, we will be tomorrow.

RECIPES

We would like to share with you some of Em's recipes. It is our hope that we will provide you with a foundation on which you can build your own. Like us, you will make some mistakes. You may not have a taste for rosemary, turmeric, or oregano, so, as Em has taught me, go slow. Never use the adage, "If a little bit is good, a whole lot more is better." All too often I have learned "a whole lot more" can ruin what could have been a delicious meal.

The recipes we have chosen to share with you are general: chicken, fish, vegetables, soups, salads, and sauces—all geared to satisfy a low-calorie diet. Please remember, your doctor may have prescribed another type of diet for you—i.e., low-sodium, low-carbohydrate, low-cholesterol. Therefore, check these ingredients carefully before using.

Em chose basic foods such as chicken and fish, simply opened her mammoth spice rack, and began doctoring—a dash here, a quarter teaspoon there, marinate this, baste that, and presto! Since Em is not writing these introductory sentences, may I say that most always her recipes were delicious. On rare occasions, however, our young gourmet's dashes became a little heavy-handed and the results devastating; hence a certain fish concoction became known as "hotsy, totsy." All it took were a few adjustments of the ingredients and "hotsy, totsy" has become one of our favorites. One of the secrets is to learn which ingredient needs to be doctored. For instance, one day, several months after I came home, I decided to take the basic vegetable soup recipe and proceed with my own doctoring. The results? Disastrous, but I was able to write Em later and proudly pinpoint why—too much basil! I *was* learning.

Let's pause for a moment to stress the importance of having the proper attitude when searching through those old favorite family hand-me-downs, the old and new cookbooks, and those mouth-watering recipes that appear throughout magazines, the daily newspaper, and sometimes even on the TV screen. Some of your prize concoctions *cannot* be doctored successfully. The best substitution in the world will rarely measure up to the real thing. Some recipes just cannot be doctored, so make up your mind now that in some things you must learn to accept second best. If bacon grease or egg yolks are bad for you, then they must go. It's as simple as that. You are what you put in your mouth.

Several helpful suggestions should make your first efforts rewarding. Begin your doctoring cautiously. We suggest starting with ¼ teaspoon of dried herbs for every four servings and ⅛ to ¼ teaspoon of spices for every four servings. For best results, add them during the last hour of cooking.

Beware of fancy combination herbs on the market. Most contain salt (sodium), some contain dehydrated vegetable fat (in otherwords, calories), some sugar (glucose, dextrose). We also caution you to check the ingredients on packaged foods: some are prepared in syrup, some water, some breaded. Some canned goods contain sugar, and most all contain salt; some are packed in oil, some in water. Here again, we cannot overemphasize: READ THE LABELS. If your salt intake has been restricted, then frozen or fresh vegetables rather than canned are a must for you unless the label clearly states no salt or sodium.

Labels that read "Diet" can be deceiving as we have mentioned. The word "Diet" generally means that the food has been processed in a different way than most. Low-sodium foods are diet foods, but some contain sugar, therefore raising the calorie count. Diet drinks have different calorie counts, depending on the brand. Be careful. *Half the calories* may not be much of a saving if the original count was high. Reading the labels will save you money, time, and frustration.

Be alert when buying salad dressings. Again, READ THE LABELS. Some diet dressings amount to around 30 calories per ounce. Usually the label states one ounce equals one tablespoon, not one ounce of *liquid* measurement. Four ounces of salad dressing, then, means 4 tablespoons, *not* ½ cup.

Try cooking fresh vegetables with the skins on for added flavor, vitamins, and nutrition. A good rubbing or washing with a vegetable brush will remove the unwanted sand and dirt, making peeling unnecessary. We also caution against overcooking. Excessive boiling will cook away most of the nutrition our bodies need.

We have listed several herb combinations that may suit your taste buds as substitutes for butter or bacon dripping when seasoning vegetables. Simply add these ingredients to the water before adding vegetables.

Scan your favorite recipes for possible substitutions. For instance, use: a non-stick pan coating instead of grease; one of the many non-caloric sweeteners for honey, syrup, or sugar; butter flavoring rather than oleo or that "high-priced spread"; sherry, rum, or brandy extract in place of wine; and skimmed or dry powdered skim milk for whole milk.

A food scale is an absolute must. Very few foods of equal size weigh the same. By the same token, raw weights vary from cooked. Be sure to weigh each food before and/or after preparation to be sure these caloric measurements agree with your prescribed diet. If your menu calls for four ounces of cooked cabbage, then weighing after cooking is called for. Four ounces of steak refers to a four ounce portion that has been cooked, deboned, and free of all visible fat. Usually a close measurement is that six ounces of raw steak equal approximately four ounces of prepared meat; six ounces of raw, skinned chicken breasts become approximately four ounces of cooked, deboned chicken. Remember, these measurements are approximates. Always weigh before serving, as a half ounce of meat, fish, or fowl can make a big difference if you are on a strict caloric diet.

135

Remember to skin all fowl before cooking. This eliminates cooking excess fat into the portion and at the same time, eliminates the temptation to eat the high-caloric skins.

If your prescribed diet allows, try several kinds of meat and fish and tailor your diet to your taste. A diet that says simply four ounces of fish gives a tremendous leeway. A calorie counter will be a great help in pinpointing what kinds of fish have the least amount of calories. Thus, most of our fish recipes were prepared using either turbot or flounder. By the same token, there are many different cuts of steak, showing a variety of caloric measurements. Both of us enjoy steak, and both react differently when steak is on our menu. For instance, an hour after Em eats steak she is ravenous. So, for her, steak can be devastating, although she loses well eating it. I, on the other hand, find steak very satisfying, but the weight does not drop. These experiences appeared in a definite pattern in our diaries.

A slow cooker is ideal for the working person and student. Simply turn it on before leaving home in the morning and dinner is ready when you return in the evening. Leaf or whole herbs and spices will produce the best flavor, and most recommended amounts should be cut in half unless using a slow-cooker recipe. Ground seasonings should be added during the last hour of cooking. Another helpful hint is to turn up the heat and uncover the cooker during the last 45 minutes to thicken the natural juices, thus eliminating the need for making gravy with flour or cornstarch.

Following are some of our recipes that will introduce you to different flavors through the use of herbs and spices. Remember, the only way to discover your likes and dislikes is to experiment. We hope that some of these recipes will satisfy your cravings as well as awaken dormant taste buds. Many cookbooks on the market today list seasonings that complement certain foods. These will further aid your own experimenting and doctoring. You're in for a treat.

Happy dieting!

BROTHER'S VEGETABLE SOUP

1 gallon chicken stock*
2 cups diced celery
2 cups diced onion
2 cups diced carrots
4 cups diced fresh tomatoes
(subtract amount of water
from chicken stock to
equal amount of tomato
water you add)

1 six-ounce can tomato paste
1 tsp. oregano
1 tsp. parsley
½ tsp. marjoram
½ tsp. thyme
½ tsp. rosemary
1 bay leaf

* To make chicken stock, use 3 pounds chicken necks, backs, and wings to 1½ gallons of water. Bring to a boil, then simmer for 2-3 hours, covered. Refrigerate until cold. Skim fat from top of bowl.

Simmer the vegetables, in just enough water to keep them from sticking, until tender. Add the stock and herbs. Add the tomato paste. Simmer, covered, for about 1 hour, or until thick. Refrigerate. Reheat to serve in 1½-cup servings.

1½ cups = 60 calories

BROCCOLI SOUPER

1¼ to 1½ lbs. fresh broccoli,
trimmed and cut up, or 2
ten-ounce packages frozen
chopped broccoli
2 thirteen-ounce cans
chicken broth (or
homemade, with fat
skimmed off)

1 medium onion
2 tbsp. diet margarine or
butter (optional)
1 tsp. salt
1-2 tsp. curry powder
dash pepper
2 tbsp. lime juice
lemon slices

Place broccoli in a large saucepan and add broth, onion, margarine, salt, curry powder, and pepper. Bring to a boil, reduce heat, and simmer, covered, 8-12 minutes or until just tender. Place half the broccoli and half the broth at a time in blender. Blend until smooth. Repeat with the other half. Stir in lime juice. Cover and refrigerate at least 4 hours. Top with lemon slices.

1½ cups soup = 30 calories

CUCUMBER SOUP

2 large cucumbers, peeled,
halved, seeded, and finely
chopped
1 qt. boiling chicken broth
3 tbsp. diet butter or
margarine (optional)

1 onion, finely chopped
¼ lb. mushrooms, sliced
1 tsp. salt
dash pepper
chopped chives, to garnish

Add cucumbers to boiling chicken broth, cover and simmer 10 minutes. Heat butter in small skillet and saute mushrooms and onions until tender (or saute them in 2 tbsp. water). Add mushrooms and onions to broth. Season with salt and pepper to taste and cook 3 minutes. Cool and chill. Place in blender and blend until creamy. Serve topped with chopped chives (fresh, if available). If desired, add 1 tsp. lemon juice to bring out the flavor after chilling.

4 servings
32 calories per serving

ZUCCHINI SOUP

1 lb. zucchini (3-4 small),
washed and sliced
1 cup chicken or beef broth
½ tsp. salt
⅛ tsp basil

⅛ tsp. thyme
⅛ tsp. marjoram
2 cups skimmed milk
1 tbsp. curry (optional)

Put zucchini, broth, and salt into a saucepan and bring to a boil. Cover and simmer gently until tender. Cool. Add basil, thyme, marjoram. Puree in blender. Stir in milk and heat (do not boil). Serve topped with cottage cheese.

1 cup = 66 calories without cottage cheese

SWISS POTATO PANCAKE

1 large raw potato, grated
1 egg white, raw
⅛ tsp. pepper
¼ tsp. salt

Mix grated potato and egg white with salt and pepper very thoroughly in a bowl. Pour onto skillet sprayed with non-stick coating. Fry over medium-high heat until golden, turning once, and serve. Garnish with a sprig of parsley and a slice of pimento, if desired.

1 serving
105 calories per serving

COLE SLAW MADELAINE

2 cups finely grated carrots
½ green pepper, diced
½ carrot, shredded
½ cucumber, peeled, seeded, and chopped
1 sweet onion, thinly sliced

2 tbsp. wine vinegar
2 tbsp. vegetable oil
2 tbsp. brown sugar substitute
1 clove garlic, minced

Combine first five ingredients in a bowl. Then add the rest of the ingredients, mix well, and let marinate in refrigerator overnight.

6 servings
66 calories per serving

TOMATO AND EGGPLANT CASSEROLE OLÉ

1 medium eggplant
1 cup chopped onion
1 clove garlic, minced
½ cup chopped celery
1 large green pepper, cut in
  strips

1 cup tomatoes, canned
¼ cup chopped parsley
1 tbsp. chopped basil
½ tsp. salt
pepper to taste
lemon wedges, for garnish

Preheat oven to 350°. Wrap eggplant in foil and cook in oven for one hour. Meanwhile, cook until wilted and slightly transparent the onion, garlic, celery, and green peppers in tomato water. Add tomatoes, parsley, and basil. Simmer mixture until slightly thickened, about 35 minutes. Remove the eggplant from the oven and open foil. Carefully split the eggplant, scoop out the flesh, and add to the casserole. Add salt and pepper. Serve the stew hot or cold with the lemon wedges.

6 servings
50 calories per serving

CABBAGE AND APPLES

½ cup shredded cabbage
¼ cup chopped apples
1 tsp. cider vinegar
1 tsp. water
artificial sweetener to taste

Cook all ingredients together over medium heat until tender, with skillet tightly covered.

1 serving
55 calories per serving

SKINNY TOMATO SAUCE

Cut up:
1 large onion
1 large green pepper
6 tomatoes (scalded and
   peeled)

Add:
3-4 garlic cloves
dash black pepper
½ tsp. oregano
3 basil leaves
artificial sweetener to taste

If tomatoes are ripe, do not add water. If not, use water to cover vegetables in saucepan. Simmer until well done, covered, about 1 hour.

4 servings
56 calories per serving

MUSTARDY SALAD DRESSING

1 jar mustard with
   horseradish
equal amount white vinegar
2 tsp. salad herbs
sweetener to taste (start with
   sweetener to equal 4 tbsp.
   sugar)

In a large jar, mix the mustard and the vinegar together. Add the salad herbs and the sweetener. Refrigerate. This dressing improves with age because the flavor of the herbs becomes stronger the longer they sit. The dressing is sharp, so don't overdo the first time you try it!

1 tbsp. = 12 calories

SAUCE FOR JERRY'S BARBECUE

4 cloves garlic
1 tsp. (equivalent) sugar
substitute
2 tbsp. tabasco
½ cup wine vinegar
½ cup soy sauce
¼ cup Worcestershire sauce

3 tbsp. diet catsup (or
Skinny Tomato Sauce, see
page 141)
½ cup water
2 tbsp. sherry extract
½ tsp. salt
dash papper

Simmer all ingredients together for 1 hour or more. Let stand in refrigerator for 1 day.

20 calories per tablespoon

COOL CUCUMBER SAUCE

1 medium cucumber
1 tbsp. vinegar
⅛ tsp. pepper
few grains cayenne
1 tsp. minced onion

Peel cucumber and chop it finely. Add remaining ingredients. Try it on cold fish.

42 calories per recipe

DILLY OF A SAUCE

½ cup skimmed milk
1 cup diet mayonnaise
1 tsp. lemon juice
¼ tsp. dill weed

Gradually stir milk into mayonnaise. Add lemon juice and dill weed. Heat on low flame, stirring occasionally until hot, 2-3 minutes.

10 calories per teaspoon

APOSTLES' FISH

¼ cup apple cider vinegar
¼ cup fish stock or water
½ cup brown sugar
   substitute
1 tbsp. prepared mustard

1 tsp. garlic powder
1 tsp. onion flakes
¼ tsp. salt
¼ tsp. pepper
1 lb. flounder filets

Marinate the fish in all the other ingredients for at least 2 hours. When ready to serve, thinly coat the fish with extra mustard, sprinkle sparsely with salt, pepper, garlic powder, and, for garnish, paprika. Broil the fish for 15 minutes. Thin filets such as flounder do not need to be turned during cooking.

Note: We asked the owner of the fish market to save the heads and tails of the fish he fileted for us, which we simmered in 1 gallon of water for many hours, making marvelous fish stock which we used in all of our fish recipes instead of water, giving a heartier flavor to the food, not at the expense of our figures!

2 servings
150 calories per serving

HOTSY TOTSY FISHY WISHY

½ cup wine vinegar
½ cup fish stock or water
1 tbsp. lemon juice
sugar substitute to equal 2
   tsp. sugar
2 tsp. dill seed
dash pepper

½ tsp. salt
½ chili pepper, finely
   chopped
1 clove garlic
1 tsp. mustard
1 lb. fish filets

Blend all ingredients but the fish together with fork. Marinate fish in mixture at least 2 hours. Spread fish with thin layer of mustard, sprinkle with salt, pepper, garlic powder, and paprika. Place fish in a shallow baking pan, pour marinade over fish, and broil for 15 minutes. Do not turn thin fish filets.

2 servings
110 calories per serving

CURRIED HADDOCK AND RICE

1 lb. haddock, 4 pieces
1 tsp. lemon juice
6 peppercorns
1 bay leaf
1 tbsp. salad oil
1 tbsp. minced onion
1 tbsp. cream of rice
1 tsp. curry powder

About 30 minutes before serving:
In medium skillet over high heat, heat 3 cups water to boiling. Reduce heat to medium-high. Add haddock, lemon juice, peppercorns, and bay leaf. Simmer, covered, 10-15 minutes or until fish flakes easily with fork. With spatula, place fish on a warm platter. Strain skillet liquid, reserving one cup.

In the same skillet, over medium heat, in oil, cook onion until limp. In small bowl, stir reserve fish liquid into cream of rice, pour into skillet, and cook until thickened, stirring frequently. Blend in curry. Pour sauce over fish and rice (½ cup = 100 calories) to serve.

4 servings
200 calories per serving without rice
300 calories per serving with ½ cup rice

SPANISH FISH

1 medium onion, minced
¼ cup minced green pepper
1 cup chopped celery
10½ oz. condensed tomato
   soup with 10½ oz. water
       or
3 cups tomato soup
½ tsp. salt
1 tsp. curry powder
1 tbsp. Worcestershire sauce

1 tsp. lemon juice
1 tsp. tarragon vinegar
1 tsp. coarse ground pepper
1 tsp. sweet basil or oregano
1 tsp. marjoram
1 tsp. chili powder
2 lbs. cooked flounder,
   flaked
2 cups cauliflower, cooked

Saute onion, green pepper, and celery in 2 tbsp. water in a pan sprayed with non-stick coating until soft, not brown. Add tomato soup (with water if condensed). Add salt, curry powder, Worcestershire sauce, lemon juice, tarragon vinegar, black pepper, basil, marjoram, and chili powder. Let stand at least 15 minutes. Place fish and 2 cups cooked cauliflower in a large bowl. Add spice mixture, and stir well. Place in a 2-quart casserole and cover. Bake in a moderate oven (350°) about 30 minutes, until heated through. Brown the top of the casserole uncovered in the broiler. Sprinkle lightly with paprika to garnish, if desired.

8 servings
4-ounce fish serving = 114 calories

CHIEF BOTTLEWASHER'S DISARMING DINNER

⅓ cup wine vinegar
⅓ cup water or fish stock
¼ cup diet catsup
1 tsp. garlic powder
1 tsp. creole seasoning
1 tsp. dill seed

1 tsp. pickling spice
1 onion, sliced, in rings
1 tsp. curry powder
½ tsp. salt
1 lb. flounder filets

Marinate fish in all ingredients for at least 4 hours, preferably overnight. Broil 15 minutes with onion rings and marinade on top. No turning necessary.

2 servings
150 calories per serving

GARDEN BOUNTY

1 tomato, peeled and
  chopped
1 cucumber, peeled, seeded,
  and chopped
1 onion (4 oz.) chopped
2 pimentos, chopped
1 clove garlic, minced
1 tbsp. vinegar

dash pepper
dash cayenne
¼ tsp. parsley, dry
½ tsp. chives
¼ tsp. oregano
½ cup tomato juice (or
  tomato soup)
8 oz. fish filets, cooked

Combine all but fish in blender. Blend until smooth on medium speed. Chill 2 hours. Cook fish (boil or broil or bake), add to sauce, and serve in bowls.

2 servings
Sauce: 55 calories per serving
Fish: 90 calories per serving

SMOKY MARINATED FISH

1 lb. fish filets
¼ cup wine vinegar
⅛ cup lemon juice
1 tbsp. grated lemon rind
½ tbsp. liquid smoke

½ tbsp. brown sugar
  substitute
¼ tsp. Worcestershire sauce
1 bay leaf
dash tabasco

Combine all ingredients except fish, and heat to boiling. Cool. Marinate filets in the mixture for 1 hour. Broil. Turn fish after 5 minutes and baste with remaining sauce. Broil until fish flakes easily, about 7-10 minutes more.

2 servings
150 calories per serving

JEAN'S STOMACH PLEASER

1 four-ounce can mushrooms
   with juice
1 large onion, sliced very
   thinly
2 stalks celery, chopped
1 green pepper, sliced thinly
⅛ tsp. garlic salt
⅛ tsp. bay leaf powder
1 lb. frozen fish filets or
   2 three-ounce ground beef
   patties

Place frozen fish or raw beef patties in non-stick skillet. Pour mushroom juice from can over meat or fish. Add herbs, then all the vegetables, and simmer over medium heat until fish flakes easily or patties are cooked as desired.

2 servings
Fish: 160 calories per serving
Meat: 120 calories per serving

ORIENTAL CHICKEN

6 chicken breasts (6 oz.
   each) split
½ cup lemon juice
¼ cup water
3 tbsp. soy sauce
¼ tsp. ground ginger
1 tsp. garlic powder

Marinate the skinned chicken in a sauce of all the other ingredients. After several hours, remove, reserving the marinade. Barbecue chicken for 30 minutes, until tender on hibachi or under the broiler. Baste frequently with marinade.

6 servings
159 calories per serving

LEMON CHICKEN

1 lemon
1 large chicken
2 large onions
3 stalks celery
4 medium carrots
1 cup mushrooms

3 bay leaves
3 peppercorns
water
1 tsp. salt
½ tsp. peppercorns

Squeeze lemon juice all over the outside of the whole chicken. Put the lemon skin inside. Put the chicken into a casserole, with whole onions, diced celery, carrots, bay leaves, and peppercorns. Cover with water to 1 inch below top of casserole. Season lightly. Cover tightly and cook at 275° for 3-4 hours. When tender, remove chicken from liquid and keep warm. Boil stock rapidly to reduce volume by one half, or less. Add mushrooms while boiling. Put stock into blender and blend until thick. Surround chicken with sauce, or pour over chicken. Garnish with sprigs of parsley.

Note: This is a good recipe with which to try new herbs. Start with a small amount of one herb, and each time, vary the herb you add and the amount. Remember, too much of a good thing can spoil the recipe altogether.

Sauce: 8 servings
15 calories per serving

ROSEMARY CHICKEN

2 fryer chickens, cut up (2
   lbs. each)
1 large onion, cut into thick
   slices
⅔ cup diet tomato catsup
⅓ cup white vinegar

1 clove garlic, minced
1 tsp. rosemary, crushed
1 tsp. salt
¼ tsp. dry mustard
1 tsp. butter flavoring

Place chicken, skin side down, in a single layer in non-stick baking pan. Top with onion slices. Mix all remaining ingredients in small saucepan. Heat just to boiling, pour over chicken. Bake at 400° for 30 minutes. Turn chicken, skin side up, baste with sauce in pan. Continue baking, basting once or twice, for 30 minutes more, until tender and well glazed.

5 servings
222 calories per serving

LAMB IN THE GARDEN

2 lbs. lamb, raw
6 medium carrots
4 medium onions
1½ cups fresh peas

2½ cups brown stock
4 tomatoes
½ tsp. marjoram
½ tsp. salt

Cut meat into cubes, arrange in a casserole with onions, whole or sliced, carrots, stock, and seasoning. Cover tightly and cook at 300° for 1½ hours. Add quartered tomatoes and peas. Leave uncovered, and cook for 30 minutes more.

Note: This is a good recipe to practice your skill with the use of herbs. Use your favorite herbs instead of marjoram, if you prefer. New herbs make new dishes!

11 servings
270 calories per serving

CUMIN-GINGER LAMB

1 tbsp. olive oil
1 tbsp. diet butter or
  margarine
2 large onions, thinly sliced
2 tbsp. chopped parsley
1 large clove garlic, minced
1 tsp. salt or salt substitute
1 tsp. ginger

1 tsp. ground cumin
½ tsp. paprika
¼ tsp. pepper
⅛ tsp. powdered saffron
2 lbs. boneless lamb, cut
  into 1″ cubes
1 tbsp. lemon juice

In a large saucepan, heat the oil and the margarine together. Stir in onions, chopped parsley, garlic, and seasonings. Add the lamb cubes, turning them constantly to coat them with onion mixture. Cover and simmer, stirring occasionally, until very tender, about 1½ hours. Remove the lamb to a serving platter, keep it warm, and cook the remaining liquid over high heat, stirring constantly, until thickened. Stir in lemon juice. Heat through. Pour over the lamb and serve.

10 servings
284 calories per serving

FRUITY LAMB CHOPS

6 three-ounce lamb chops
1 cup canned drained
   pineapple (use water
   packed)
1 tsp. grated orange rind

2 tbsp. finely chopped mint
½ tsp. dry ginger
½ cup pineapple juice
2 tbsp. apple cider vinegar

Place lamb chops in a shallow pan sprayed with non-stick coating, and mix the crushed pineapple, orange rind, mint, and ginger in a separate bowl. Pour this mixture over the lamb chops and bake at 350° for 45 minutes to 1 hour. Add ½ cup pineapple juice heated with the vinegar, and serve.

6 servings
209 calories per serving

BREADED VEAL (OR FISH) CUTLET

½ cup cream of rice
½ tsp. pepper
½ tsp. dry mustard

juice of half a lemon
4 veal cutlets or fish filets

Rub each cutlet or filet with lemon. Dip each into mixture of cream of rice, pepper, and dry mustard, and fry in a pan sprayed with a non-stick coating, or broil to desired doneness.

4 servings
Veal (4 oz.): 145 calories per serving
Fish (4 oz.): 110 calories per serving

LAMB WITH MUSHROOMS

2 lbs. lamb. (3 oz. cooked per
   serving)
3 cups mushrooms
2 large or 8 small onions
4 medium carrots

1½ cups fresh beans
1⅓ cups fresh peas
½ tsp. salt
pepper to taste

Cut meat into cubes. Put into pan with water and sliced or whole carrots. Bring to a boil and simmer steadily for 1 hour. Then add the mushrooms, beans, peas, and seasoning. Simmer for 45 minutes.

11 servings
264 calories per serving

T.V. TIDE-OVER

1 heaping teaspoon chocolate
   flavored skim milk powder
1 tsp. decaffeinated instant
   coffee
artificial sweetener to taste

Add hot water and stir. Scrumptious!

**1 serving
30 calories**

SIP 'N' STUDY

1 heaping teaspoon
   decaffeinated instant
   coffee
dash cinnamon
artificial sweetener to taste
skimmed milk

To coffee, cinnamon, and sweetener, add boiling water until cup is ½ to ¾ full. Add milk and fill to the top.

**1 serving
25-30 calories per serving**

EPILOGUE

We offer no miracles, only the tools that will help you adhere to your own dietary needs. We cannot delineate why dieting is necessary for you, nor can we supply the necessary determination. Before you can successfully begin any dietary program there are several very pertinent questions to be explored. "Where am I going?" "For what purpose is my life right now?" "Why am I living?"

It wasn't until we were able to honestly see ourselves, not as we would like others to see us but as we really are, that we were able to begin swimming against the tide of our lives which had been carrying us further downstream into obesity. It's not good enough to say "I ought to change my way of living" or "I wish I could change my habits." Only when you are able to look in the mirror and say, "I've had it, I'm disgusted with the way I look; it's time I did something about it, right now," and only then, will a long-range diet program be successful. Only then will this book be of help to you.

Each of us hit rock bottom twice. We are not ashamed to admit this because we have learned from our mistakes. Both of us initially answered our own soul-searching questions and were open to the therapy that provided the incentive to reach goal. And we did.

However, within three months after reaching goal, the scale began escalating for both of us. Why? The answer was not easily forthcoming and we really had to put forth serious thought. What we finally arrived at was this: We both had reached our immediate goal and simply did not substitute another. We no longer had that necessary something to work toward. Instead of looking toward something positive, we were looking for a pat on the back to feel accepted as normal human beings by our associates. We no longer had the motivating force that is so necessary to carry us through each day. Once again, we had no goal, no purpose. We were merely existing as before we began this program. The challenge had been met and won, and we relaxed.

This second weight gain made us realize that dieting for the sake of losing weight alone is not enough. Initially, this can be sufficient motivation, but now we knew we could be successful. We had proved this. What we lacked this second time was the driving force, the determination to succeed, another goal. The behavioral therapy aspect, we found, cannot be put aside once goal is reached. This book then provides therapy not only for dieting but for living as well. Once goal is reached, the only thing that changes is the goal itself. The assertiveness training and the newly established habits and behaviors remain and new purposes in life provide the impetus to maintain the structured daily living this book teaches.

Once we understood there is more to life than merely existing from day to day, we individually searched for a purpose to make our life meaningful. Once we had again looked in the mirror and again asked those same questions, we were able to successfully begin our dieting once more. This time, as we neared our goal weight, we found we could successfully incorporate other goals. And as we continue down life's road, our therapy provides the sturdy foundation so necessary in building a better us.

So to be and remain successful, there are four necessary steps to follow:
1. Take a good look at yourself as you really are. No dodging.
2. Find a purpose, a goal to work toward that will provide the motivation and determination for success.

153

3. Follow the guidelines we have detailed in our book explaining how, through behavioral therapy, success can be achieved.
4. Don't stop just because one goal has been accomplished. As one goal is realized, seek another to maintain your purpose and zest in living.

These are the steps by which we daily build a better us.

INDEX

A

Activities, 34, 42–46, 95, 120–21
Aggression, 39–41, 45, 53, 112
Anxiety, 52–55, 60
Assertion, 39–41, 45, 53, 56, 67, 69–70, 78,
    89–91, 112, 122

B

Boredom, 42–43, 46, 51, 132

C

Charts, daily, 25–26, 29
Communication, 41, 116, 118, 122–123,
    130–31
Companionship, 47, 65–6, 77–8, 101
Comparison, 54, 66
Compliments, 71, 73–4
Confidence, 53, 78, 101
Contracts, 48–9, 80, 83–4, 91, 113, 123
Criticism, 75–6

D

Diaita, 63
Diaries, 35, 40–1, 136
Diuretics, 32
Doctor's consultations, 17–19, 30, 65–6, 78, 96, 131

E

Exercise, 18, 26–8, 51, 100

F

Fasting, 62–3
Fear, 71–4
Friendship, 45, 65–6, 77–8, 101, 122

G

Goals, 35, 78, 101–2, 127, 131
Grocery shopping, 60, 79–80, 110, 113, 126
Guilt, 45, 49, 61, 101

H

Habits, 34–5, 97
Hobbies, 43, 114
Honesty, 41, 117, 123, 127–8, 131–132
Hor's d'oeuvres, 69
Hypertension, 31–2

J

Jealousy, 76–8, 116

L

Leftovers, 123–4, 126–7
Loneliness, 46, 132

M

Maintenance, 93–7, 109–14, 115–32
Meal scheduling, 22–3

Menues, 109–10, 117–18
Monotony, 42–3, 46

N

Non-assertion, 39–41, 45, 72, 76–7
Normal eating, 78
Normal looking, 75, 91–2

P

Personal appearance, 64–6, 73
Photographs, 17, 19, 101
Physical activity, 26–30
Physical examination, 17–19
Planning and preparation, 79–82, 91, 97,
    120–21

R

Recipes, 110–11, 114, 133–51
Restaurants, 54–5, 57, 60
Rewards, 35, 41, 46, 117
Role playing, 53–4

S

Scale, 25, 65, 117–19
Self, 36, 69–70, 132
Self-confidence, 53–4, 78, 101–02
Self-control, 45, 51, 63, 90
Sharing, 132
Signs, 20–22, 36
Slow cookers, 136

T

Temptation, 44–45, 99–100, 126–27
Tension, 46, 59–63, 72, 112, 115–117

U

Unstructured eating, 48, 50–51, 100–02

V

Vanity behaviors, 65, 73, 105

W

Walking, 18, 28–30, 32, 50, 100, 120
Walking apparel, 27
Weight gain, 32–33, 59
Will power, 45, 51, 63, 127